Excision

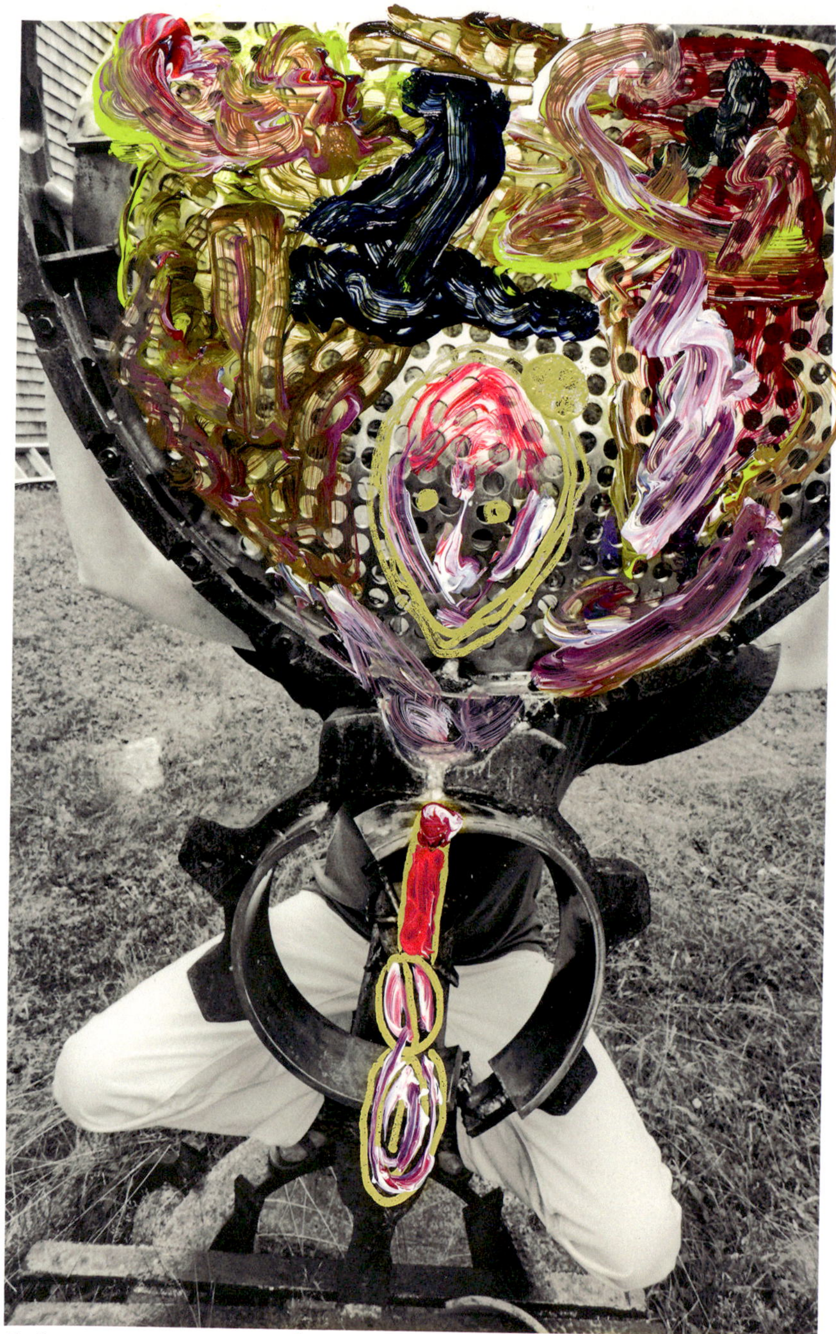

THE UNKNOWN 06 SEPT 09

Excision

Studio George Steeves

2017

Dedicated to

Ingrid Kristina Jenkner

and the doctors, nurses, technicians, and staff
of the Nova Scotia Cancer Centre at
the Victoria General Hospital, Halifax
&
The Victorian Order of Nurses

Prelude

This is a recounting in words and photographs of love, a late-in-life marriage, and advanced cancer. The events span less than two years, start to finish (2009–2010).

Ingrid Jenkner and I, George Steeves, were firmly in love by early 2008. We met in the process of mounting an exhibition of my work at the Mount Saint Vincent University Art Gallery, where Ingrid is director. At the time Ingrid was 53 and I was 65. Ingrid was a widow, having lost her spouse to a heart attack five years before. I had been living alone for the past eleven years. Both of us had two previous marriages. Our wedding took place on 23 December 2008 in Toronto in the presence of Ingrid's German parents. Each of us owned a house, Ingrid's in the country and mine in the city of Halifax. The shuttling between them was highly impractical. Ingrid sold her Lake Echo house and all its contents. She and her cat moved in with me in July 2009. Five weeks later Ingrid was diagnosed with advanced colon cancer. This narrative picks up at that point.

A compounding series of life collisions then almost simultaneously ensued. Marrying late in life is risky, just because of the inevitable baggage and set ways carried by both parties. Sudden cohabitation after years of solitude is a steep climb. Lay on top of those anticipated difficulties a cancer diagnosis and the difficulties become almost overwhelming. Circumstances such as these understandably produce extreme behaviour, for some of which no one is ever proud. There is no possible preparation for such a baptism of fire. Notwithstanding, this is a record of romance, of love, and of lust in the maelstrom of a cancer treatment that cheated death.

The photographs were made with purely documentary intentions at Ingrid's invitation. The harsh, sometimes cruel, raw images did not reflect my survivor's recollective sensibility. Only by over-painting them could I administer the necessary corrective. The paint is not intended to obscure; it tells the truth slant. The text is in a diaristic form because it is a slightly cleaned up version of minutely hand-printed annotations I made on a daily basis.

> Tell all the truth but tell it slant—
> Success in Circuit lies
> Too bright for our infirm Delight
> The Truth's superb surprise
> As Lightning to the Children eased
> With explanation kind
> The Truth must dazzle gradually
> Or every man be blind—
>
> —EMILY DICKINSON, *#1263*

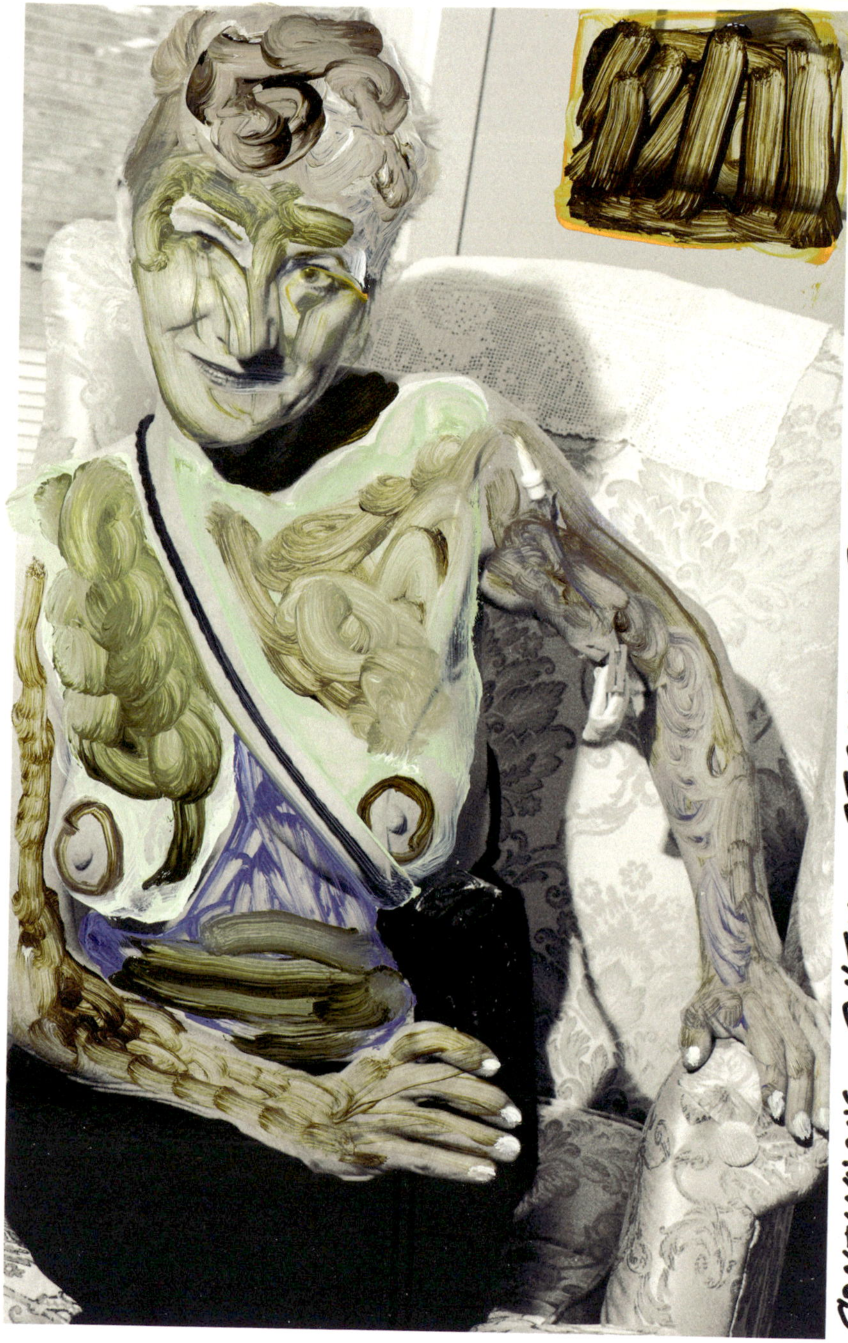

CONTINUOUS CHEMO BEGINS 2009 SEPT 14

On the Topic of Cancer

(from contemporaneous notes)

AUGUST 2009

1&2: IJ's first weekend as a resident of Fortress Tangmere. This will be an arduous period of adjustment for us both. I have lived alone for the past eleven years and IJ has recently sold her own home and most of her possessions to move in with me. Fucked brutally & balls-deep on Sunday morning in the teak bed. IJ left the kitchen in a total mess after just making soup.

3: IJ, 'Bull in a China Shop', as she plows her way into making space in the house for herself and the cat. This is reasonable and expected. The house has been transformed over the years into a photographic studio and production facility with only minimum living accommodations.

4: IJ clogged downstairs toilet with cat litter and departed for the gallery without saying a proper goodbye. I took IJ to my GP, Dr. Somers @ 2:45p for a check-up, her country GP is incompetent. Somers digitally examined her anus in front of me and discovered traces of blood. After leaving the room and thinking about it, he made an appointment for her with a surgeon for a full colorectal examination.

5: IJ joined me in bed for mid-morning intercourse and left for a gallery event @ noon. Cat exploring the yard. Wrote letter to Chester Pelkey about his ideas for a book about the *Excavations* series.

6: Solid letter to Geoffrey Simmins (Calgary) and a compendium letter to Angela Lane (England). Ordered used Hasselblad metal case to store unused cameras. Cat on the rampage, attacked livingroom carpet.

7: Nightmares about events at the Bedford Institute of Oceanography, my erstwhile employer. Letter to Martha Langford & Donigan Cumming in Montreal. Sorrowful phone message from ex-girlfriend Miss Heller. Calm has come to me from fatigue and worry, I suppose.

8: Sexless Saturday. Shopped together for bathroom fixtures. Worked on downstairs bathroom. IJ very restless, walked to store for cigarettes. Cooked fresh tuna steaks and yellow beans.

9: Waves of serious black depression, easily masked from IJ. Walked together in Hemlock Ravine. Had the camera but didn't use it. Hung IJ's personal art collection in the house.

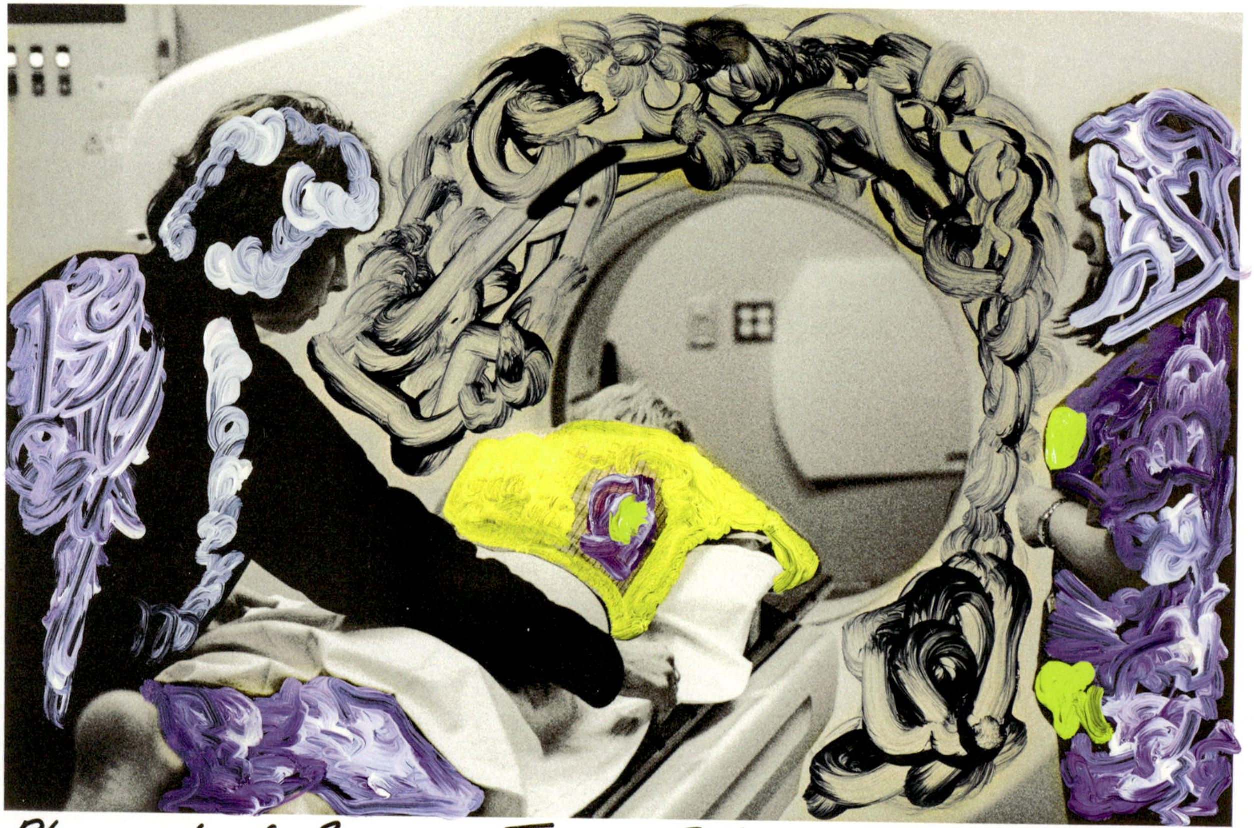

Placement of Radiation Target Tattoos Sept 2009

10: Read e-mail from Miss Heller who was shocked by encountering the joint IJ & GS telephone announcement message. She was never allowed to live here. Depressing and purposeless day. Cooked German burgers for supper.

11: Diplomatic but truthful letter to Miss Heller regarding the 'Woofer', the parasitical loser ex-husband that she never has escaped. Conversed with NSR (2nd wife) who has lots of theatrical costume work in Toronto. Bad night in bed with IJ, up @ 3:30a in wretched mood.

12: To Gaudet Optical for Zeiss spectacle lenses, parked outside Miss Heller's old place. Very strange morning. Seismic shifts in everything shaking me to the core.

13: Lyrical letter to Geoffrey Simmins. Booked into Shaw's Hotel on PEI for memorial meet up with sister Judith & husband Trent. Wrote chatty letter to IJ's parents.

14: Splendid sex @ dawn. Metro Burner @ 8:30a for annual furnace maintenance. IJ has been recalled about an anomalous mammogram on the 21st. Cleaned the house.

15: Woke with purple-headed throbbing erection. Purchased two new reading lamps for the house. A near-serious car accident in the Superstore parking lot. Nerves very bad. Miss Heller is suffering, and not in silence. IJ is aggressively punching through into Tangmere.

16: Solid quality sex @ 3:30a, then usual broken sleep. Made German-style potato salad. Took IJ to the sacred tide pool, rough-terrain hiking, fell twice, then the ritual of bathing of the genitals in ice-cold seawater.

17: Garon for coffee, always good to see my old colleague and shipmate. Appointment with my financial advisor at the bank, @ 2:00p, a slick and slippery little fuck. Stiff and sore, banged up, and lame from yesterday's falls near the tide pool.

18: Very hot +32°C. Started letters to Peter Schwenger and Geoffrey Simmins. Still very sore from falling on the rocks near Peggy's Cove.

19: Early morning quality intercourse. Nerves bad today. How strange to be alive—I should be gone—tidying up my financial affairs first though—well, some at least.

20: IJ (Didy) and the cat (Bulger) suddenly very happy here. Shopped summer vegetables. Black Hasselblad case arrived. Miss Heller near psychotic at my silence.

21: 2nd level mammography at Dixon Centre @ 11:15a. Took IJ to the appointment in the VG complex, still richly symbolic after almost 24 years since my suicide attempt of 1985. Didy stalwart and brave.

22: *Lohengrin* from the Met. Hurricane watch. Didy fucked with elan twice in 12 hours. Sawed down broken tree in backyard. IJ still pushing for her space and place. My ex-wife's (NSR) last visit to Tangmere was 22 August 2005, so IJ has a clean slate.

23: Hurricane Bill is upon us. Low atmospheric pressure (948 MB) is hard on one's head. Didy tearful and weepy in the afternoon. Maybe she has regrets—or fears, more likely. Hard night with IJ, slept in both beds badly, cat is tormenting me. Nerves very bad. This always happens when disaster is imminent. Hurricane quite mild, some broken tree limbs about the yard.

24: IJ slept downstairs alone but then put the cat out @ 1:30a and got in bed with me and we slept rather well. Prolonged teasing sex in the morning. Spent the day cleaning & trying to make the house right.

25: Terrible night, attacked by the fucking cat; she's dominating the house. Nightmare: Aubrey & Judith (my father and sister) throwing me out of Tangmere & me begging them to let me stay in the darkroom. IJ announced that she was staying 'home' today. After a night of broken sleep—now what?

26: Tired and sore from yesterday's yard work. Lunch with Miss Heller, 1st encounter in 6 weeks. I am doing the best I can to keep her from another manic-depressive psychotic episode. As is always the case with her, I was upset and had painful stomach cramps. The manipulative and accusatory Miss Heller also very upset and pathetic.

27: Wonderful clear cool dry day. Cleaned the house. Didy received her first bill for common household expenses. She came home early from the gallery to begin the purging process of her gastrointestinal track for tomorrow's rectal invasive procedure.

28: Colonoscopy @ 7a Victoria General Hospital. In the waiting room for those who accompany people being examined, there is an unmarked black telephone on one of the columns. It rang and I picked up the receiver before anyone else could get to it. The call was for me, "The doctor wants to speak to you and your wife." My heart sank while I tried to remain outwardly calm and steady. Didy has advanced colon cancer. Dr. Jamieson, "You have cancer and your life will never be the same." He outlined the standard of care, a treatment regime of MRI, radiation, chemotherapy, then radical surgery, and then heavier chemo. And it's a beautiful warm late summer day! I drove home, both of us so silent, me trying not to crash the car, and wondering "What has befallen me, us? Is Didy going to die? Like this? So soon?"

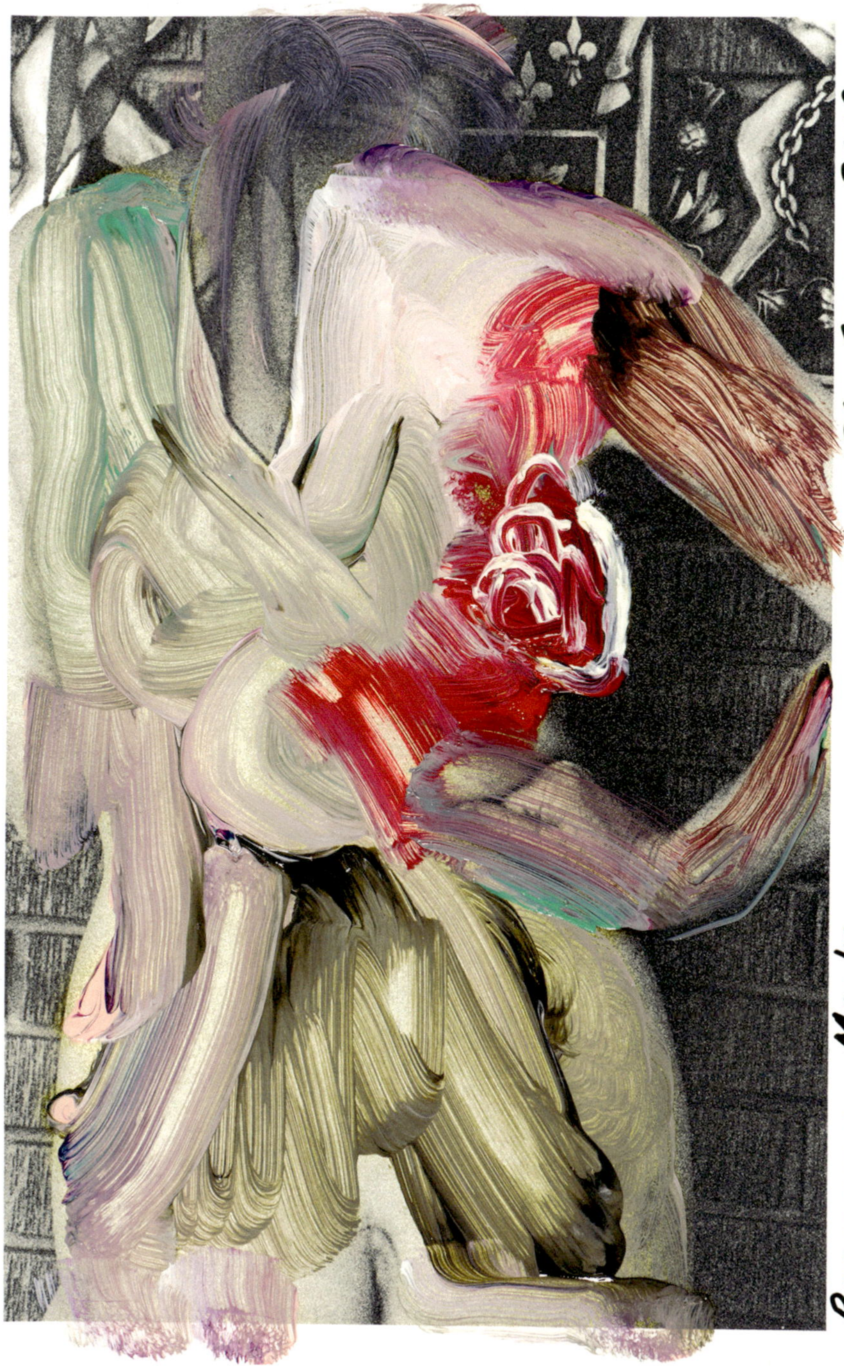

Radiation Marks 26 Sept 2009

29: Opera *Der Freischütz*, a very good Met performance. We witnessed this work at Staatsoper Berlin 2007. Trying to go on as best we can. Feeling intense tenderness for Didy. Slowly the enormity of it all is sinking in. Cooked together most of the day & didn't drink too much.

30: Party at Prof. Randi Warne's @ 5p. Didy did not tell her parents about the diagnosis on the scheduled Sunday morning phone call. She was joyful at the barbeque & I was lost in my head, unable to shake off the dark mood.

SEPTEMBER 2009

1: Drawing up a new will providing for IJ—Jeffrey Blucher @ 10a Purdy's Wharf, lawyer of wills & estates. Arose together @ 3a so IJ can work on an essay. Didy very upset, tearful, and visibly frightened.

2: We slept peacefully on wine and Valium. Another lost day devoted to internal thoughts. Beautiful days these are, so sadly so, and the pet crows have disappeared.

3: IJ came home @ noon to work on her essay. But we started on the whiskey @ 2:30p & drank too much. She wants me to photographically document her cancer treatment. This truly surprised and delighted me. It's a dangerous thing to attempt; I know that.

4: Slightly hungover and very sad. Didy looked so old and worn this morning. Ordered 35mm T-Max film from B+H in New York. Long phone conversation with Martha and then Donigan. Also phoned Valerie Dean, long time friend and model who recently moved to Halifax from Montreal.

5: Opera *Die Zauberflöte*. Didy broke the news to her sister Karin in a long whiskey-fuelled conversation. Also she spoke to Martha in Vermont. Then she told me about the $80K judgement against her for legal damages resulting from an automobile accident. The action has been pending for 3 or 4 years.

6: Lunch with artist Peter Walker near Blandford. Poignant memories of his artist wife Nancy Edell who died not so long ago of cancer. Strangely, IJ was silent re. her cancer diagnosis. Began shooting IJ.

7: Rough night with Didy, almost unbearably restless—poor dear. Today bright and cool. IJ worked on her essay & I cooked and cleaned. She's not a very co-operative house mate.

8: Didy for bone density x-ray measurement @ 1:30p, as if such would matter now. IJ up @ 1:00a to work on essay, a foolish decision. I printed 30+ postcards for the Xmas mailout while Didy smoked and wrote. Not a very loving creature at the moment, but I'm full of warmth and attachment for her anyway.

9: Up @ 5a, Didy on essay while I printed some disturbing Xmas postcards of the despicable Tim Dunn. Very nervous & troubled. DVDs of theatre performance arrived from Jo Lechay & Eugene Lion, supplemental to the *Entertainment* photo series. Cat injured her paw. The Tory gov't has killed the nascent National Portrait Gallery of Canada.

10: Didy to my dentist, Dr. Russel MacSween @ 9:30a. CT (computed tomography) scan at Victoria General main floor @ 12:30p. Another emotional visit to the hospital redolent of 1985 memories. The days are exceptionally beautiful.

11: Woke with an attack of gout. Letter to Geoffrey Simmins. Talked to ex-girlfriend Ellen Pierce whose book of verse is coming out soon. Talked to Miss Heller, who won't acknowledge that by spreading her hairy legs for Jason Holt while I was at my mother's funeral, she killed our relationship. I had previously ignored lesser dalliances with Bob Burgess. Suddenly it's too awfully quiet here.

12: Dvořák's opera *Rusalka*. Trip to PEI cancelled. A very troubled day indeed. Didy lashing out at me. Then I decided that I should unilaterally inform her father Wolfgang of her diagnosis. I did that, and it did clear the air, then talked twice to sister Karin to close the Jenkner family loop. We consumed 40 oz. of whiskey today.

13: A troubled and frightening night, woke up @ 11:00p angry and alone. Then had succulent intense sex with IJ @ 2a. She talked to her 'elders' mid-morning. They were not overly pleased that it was I who delivered the bad news. Good loving day with Didy.

14: Took IJ to GP, Dr. Patrick Somers @ 11:30a. Then to the VG for marathon session (1:45p to 4:30p) with the sexy chemo nurse practitioner, Donna Grant, whom we christened 'Blue Eyes'. Didy and I now coming to appreciate the enormity of all this. Cleaned the house upstairs.

15: Appointment with radiation specialist, Dr. Maureen Nolan, @ 1:00 Victoria Bldg. 11th floor, Cancer Centre. A better tho' for me a terrible day—alone in one mind & together in another.

16: Erratic sleep. Didy very jittery and occasionally tearful. Printed 45 postcards of 'Astrid and the Octo' for the Xmas mailout. Lovely autumnal day.

17: Mail from IJ's mother & Marjorie Simmins. Responded to Ellen's nosey and unappreciated inquiry re. Didy's condition.

18: Visions of a maimed Didy. Letters to Geoffrey and Chester Pelkey. Conversation with LFH. Took Lebanese roll-ups to MSVU Gallery for lunch with IJ. Much whiskey consumed this evening.

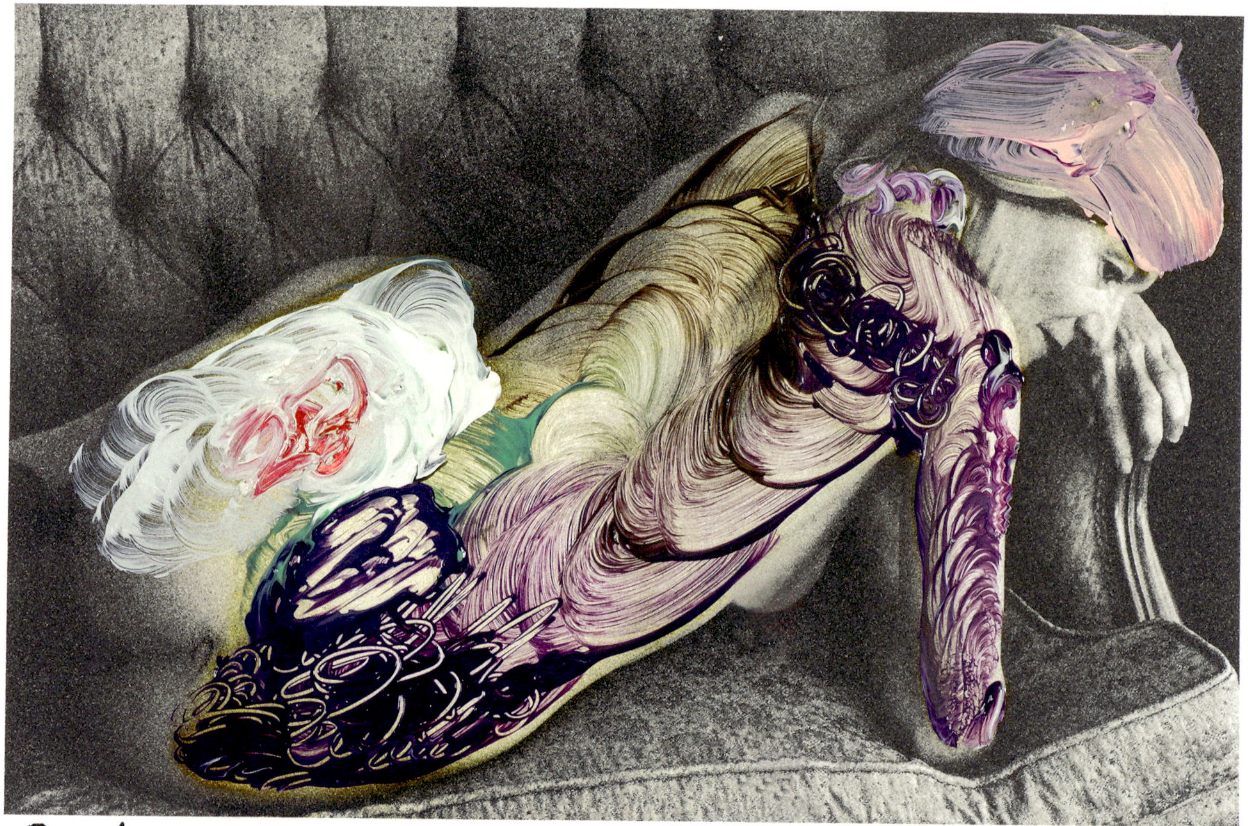

Odalisque 26 Sept 2009

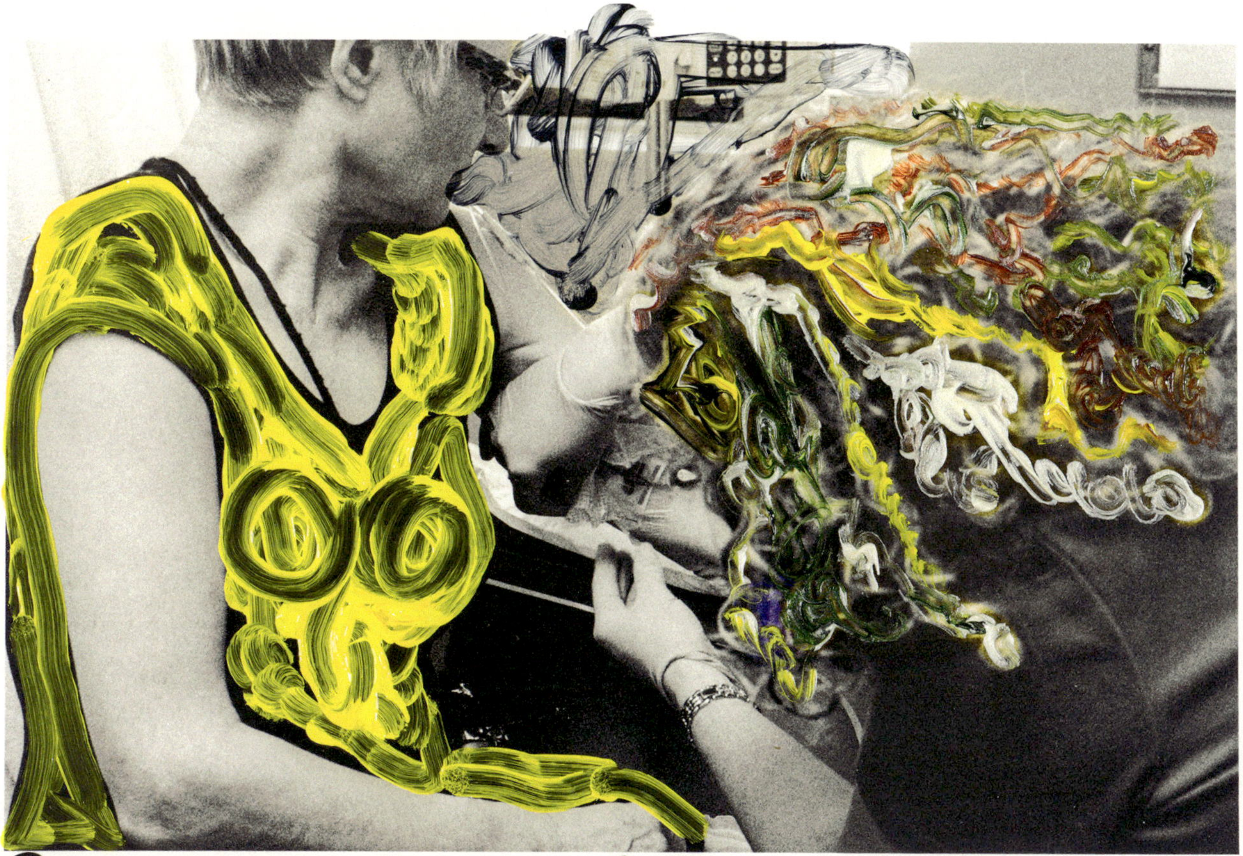

PERIPHERALLY INSERTED CENTRAL CATHETER

SEPT 2009

19: Sex for breakfast. Elders called @ 9:15a. A usual Saturday but especially tender & caring, the weather lovely, sky grey & then white by turns. The old familiar September desire to die.

20: Sex before espresso. Didy looking stricken. Soft autumnal day. Shot a test roll of film with Didy. Reviewed new will now that I know about the $80K legal judgement pending against IJ.

21: Very stressful day, upset that doorbell stopped working. Could not focus on anything. Wrote to my lawyer about Didy's legal woes.

22: Autumnal Equinox. Long talk with Donigan, told him everything. Installed new doorbell.

23: Very angry with Didy re. her selfish inconsiderate ways, but this passes. Made 22 photocards (fellatio-themed) for the real Photoland bastards on the Xmas mailout list. Calmed down and made a good supper.

24: Talk with Marjorie & LFH. Didy worked at home this afternoon. Printed Lisbon postcards.

25: Sensitive sex after coffee. Radiation Centre @ 1:45p, CAT scan simulator for mapping areas to be irradiated and tattoos applied for location repeatability. Photographed in the CAT scan facility. Very emotional day. Didy almost overcome by the mechanics of cancer treatment.

26: Opera Strauss' *Die schweigsame Frau* (The Silent Woman). Photographed Didy nude with tattoos. Shopped at Pete's for comestibles as if everything in the world was new. Worked in backyard. Cooked swordfish with Australian red sparkling wine.

27: 24th Anniversary of my 1985 suicide attempt. Languorous sex mid-morning. Talked to Wolfgang. Didy happy in her delightful way. Later she was in pain with constipation caused by a bowel obstruction.

28: Small kitchen fire caused by a felt trivet on bottom of kettle. Spent most of the day cleaning every surface & item in the kitchen. Didy very happy because MSVU President, Alexa McDonough, offered her reassurances re. IJ's job guarantee while on sick leave.

29: Didy to dentist @ 3:40p. Didy's constipation has passed. Made chicken noodle soup. Didy very upset by the case of Diana Nemiroff and her dying husband in Ottawa. Called sister Judith, a senior public health nurse, to intercede.

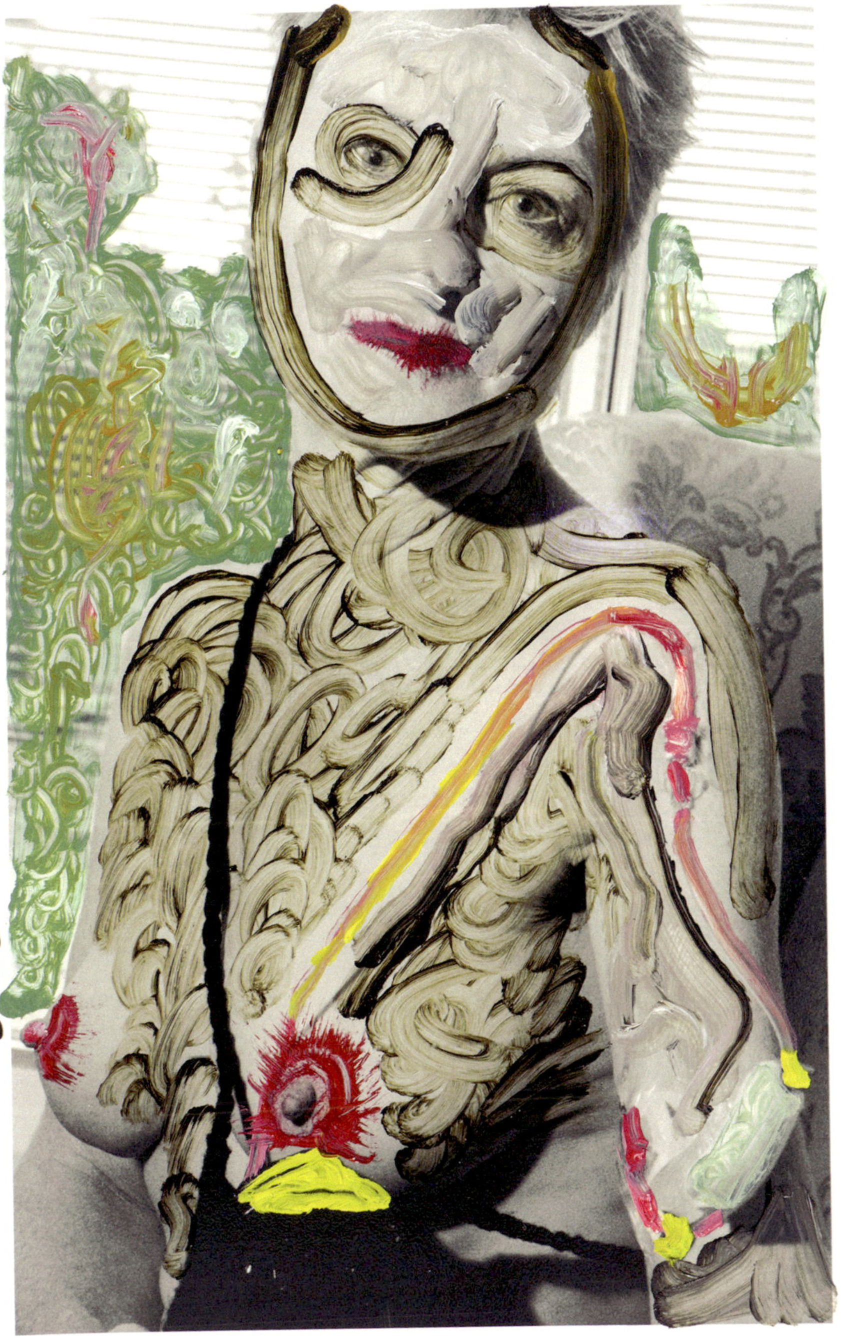

5-FLL PICC LINE SEPT 2009

30: Marjorie Simmins and Silver Donald Cameron @ 10a. Marjorie brought cooked food. Bulger, the cat, playfully teased their dog through the windshield of their car. Great visit, though it's exhausting to explain all that is happening. Spent the afternoon in emotional recovery.

OCTOBER 2009

1: Didy to dentist @ 10a for second appointment in dental rehabilitation. Geoffrey Simmins correspondence. Very nervous this afternoon. Glad to see Didy after work, felt close to her.

2: Garon for coffee @ 10a and a long and thorough conversation. Garon has a positive and practical life view that is always helpful to me. Phoned Miss Heller who is spending the weekend with Jason Holt and has communicated with Astrid. Talked with perfidious sister Judith.

3: Opera Strauss' *Ariadne auf Naxos*. Beautiful autumnal day. To Mills Bros. to buy Didy a new winter coat for Xmas, a lovely black wool Italian. Some shooting in the afternoon.

4: Talked to Wolfgang, we are warming to each other. I'm not at ease on the phone because I can't see the face I'm talking to, and Wolfgang is a man of few words. Tested Nikon F4 smart flash. Photographed Didy in bathtub. Cooked a Thanksgiving-style Sunday dinner.

5: IJ's insane mother's birthday. Problem with getting Didy on the Pensioner's Dental Plan. Very nervous & depressed. Where will life lead now?

6: Loving morning slow ritualized intercourse. Photographed a large spider on the deck. Printed 42 images from Lisbon for Xmas mailout. Contacted Linda with the news—she will come to see us at Tangmere next week.

7: Double 10a appointment with GP Dr. Somers. Cooked fancy German casserole. IJ fighting with university administration about hiring her temporary replacement.

8: Letters to Geoffrey Simmins and Angela Lane. Hospital called to set up schedule of appointments for next week's initiation of therapy. Battle continues with MSVU re. letter guaranteeing continuing employment.

9: IJ to appeal directly to the university president and involve Silver Donald Cameron. Didy successful in obtaining assurances from Alexa McDonough. IJ learned today of the suicide of artist and pedagogue Gerald Ferguson two days ago by a revolver shot to the head. IJ and Susan Gibson-Garvey had coffee with him just a few days before, with no indication of what he had long been planning. Phoned painter Susanna Heller (sister of Miss Heller) in NYC about 'Jerry' Ferguson, who taught and mentored Susanna at NSCAD.

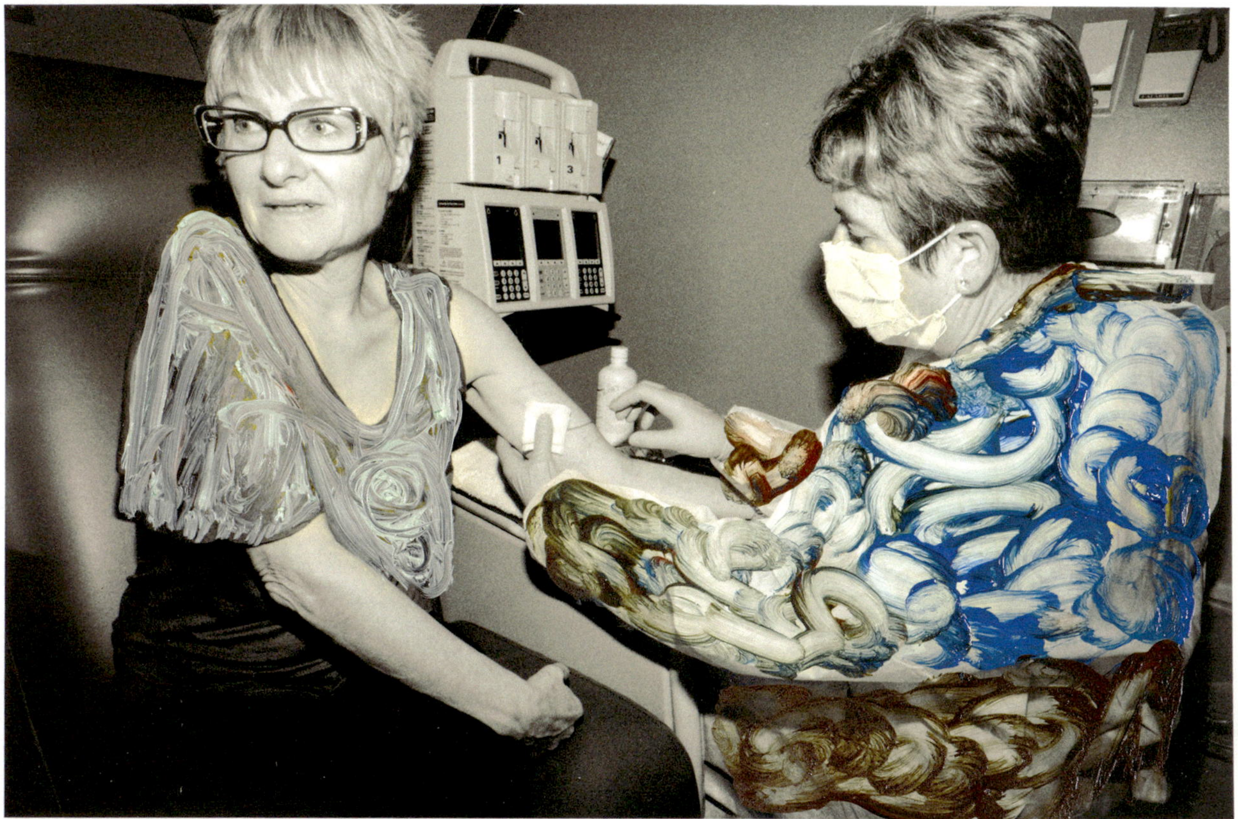

CATHETER INSERTION 13 OCT 2009

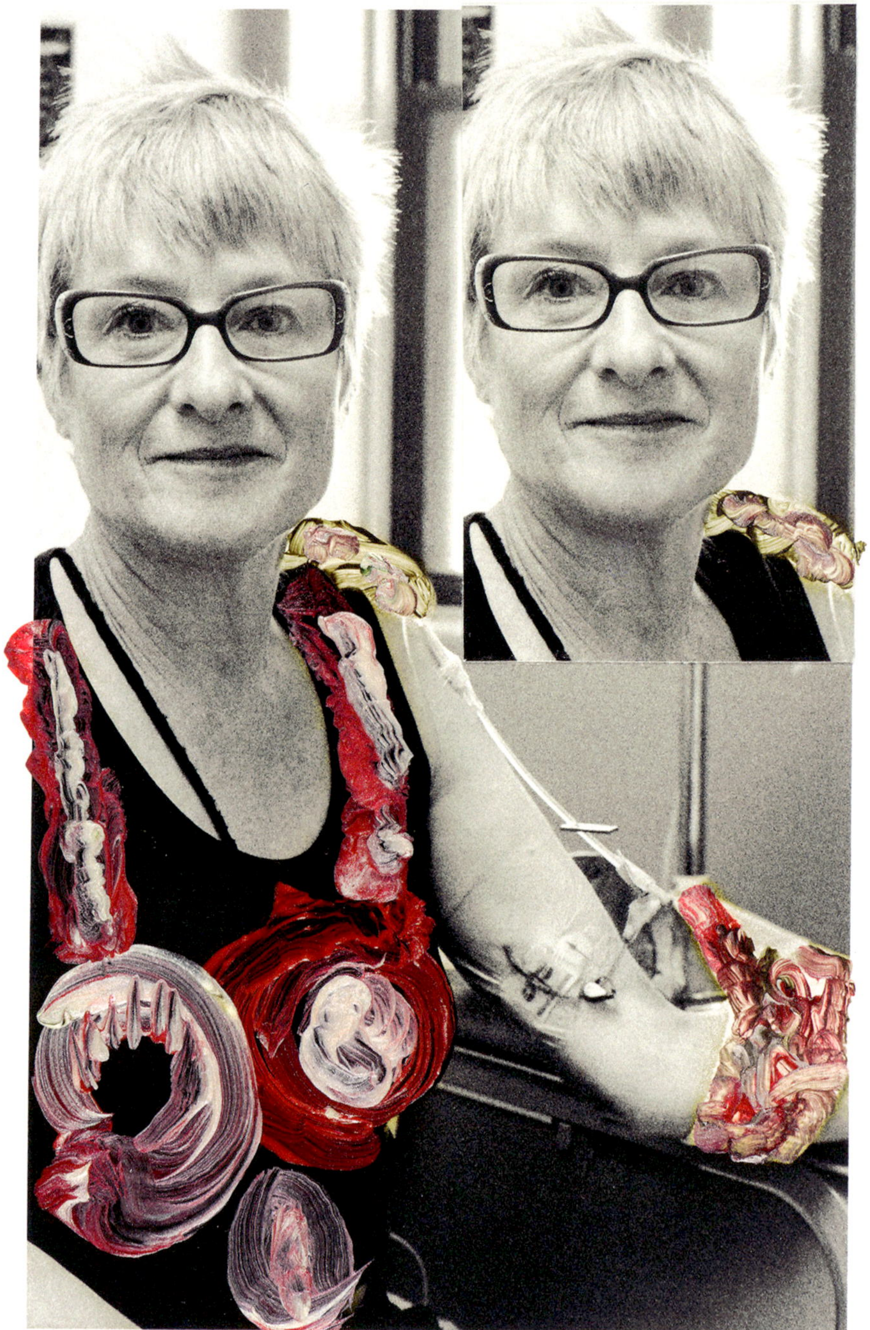

SEPTEMBER 2009 VICTORIA GENERAL

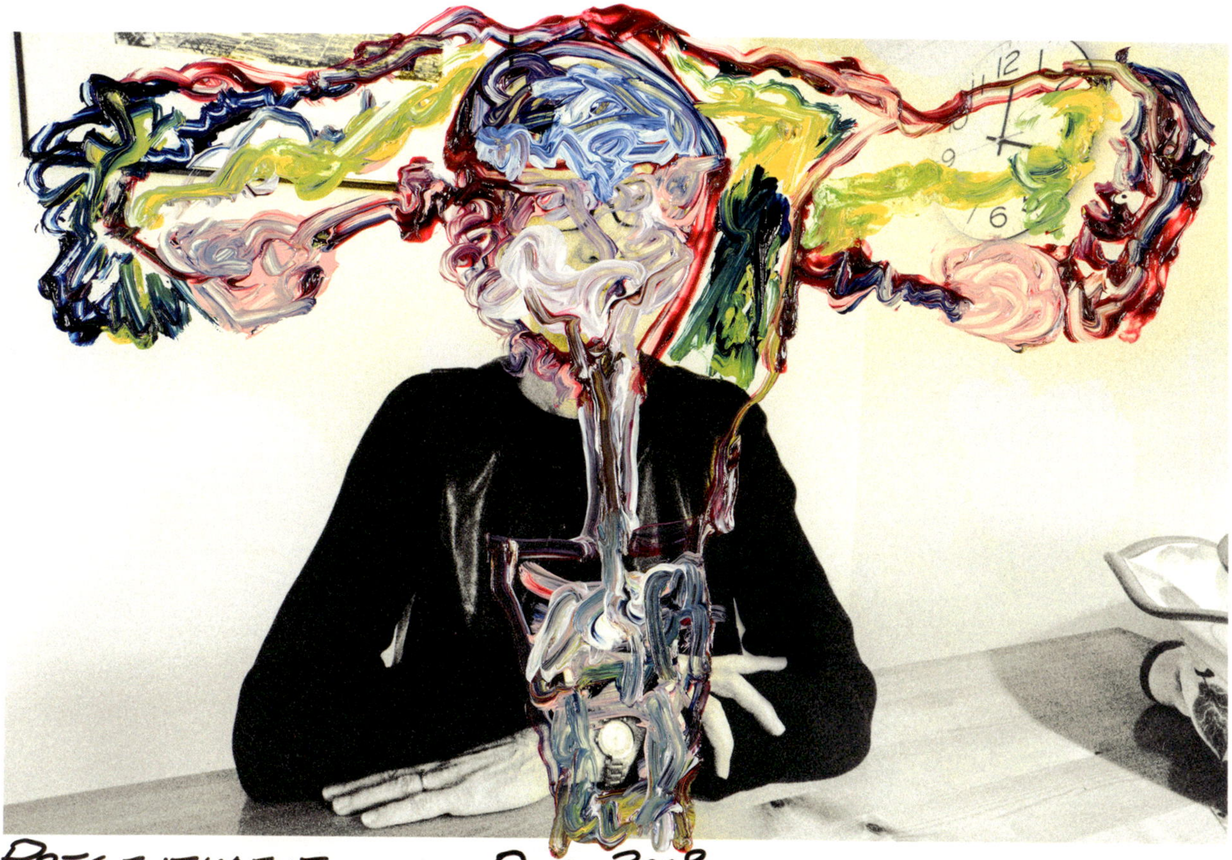

PRESENTIMENT   OCT 2009

10: Opera *Madama Butterfly*. Up @ 4a for cigs on the deck followed by vigorous sex. Didy in a good mood after her last day at the gallery yesterday until the treatment is over sometime next spring. Emotional afternoon beset by memories of Thanksgivings past when my Mum was alive and NSR was still here. The striped maples are a glorious yellow riot in the backyard.

11: Elders quite ill with bad colds. Enjoyable Thanksgiving dinner at Fran Dorsay's. Very touched that Peggy MacKinnon deposited apple pie near the front door.

12: Thanksgiving Day, very cold and sunny. Peaceful and colourful autumn day. IJ's sister Karin called for a long conversation. Fooled around with old Leica M4 but could not muster the desire to make any pictures.

13: Disturbed sleep but woke focussed and on alert. PICC line installation @ 9a (peripherally-inserted central catheter), a tube running up the left arm and into the chest cavity for the continuous administration of 24/7 chemotherapy. Didy looked terrified during the procedure which I photographed. Excellent medical staff. Didy greatly relieved when it was over.

14: Chemo bottle installation and first radiation treatment @ 3:45p. Bathed and shampooed Didy for first time so as to protect the butterfly catheter and chemo supply bottle. I haven't physically cared for another since I saw my parents out. Cold day, threatening to snow.

15: Check out of PICC line and radiation treatment #2 @ 9:15a. Exhausting day, another reality accepted. Upbeat letter from Geoffrey and note from Nicolas Comeau in MTL.

16: Radiation #3 @ 2:30p. Shopped for needed household items: toilet seat, doorbell, nightlight, muffin tin, and chopping board. Cheering visit from Peggy Mac.

17: Opening at MSVU Gallery of show *Somewhere along the Line*. Didy did not officiate, only the 2nd time in all her years there. Didy not well today, chemo and radiation fatigue.
Saturday shopped alone then made a pot of nourishing beef and vegetable soup. Didy slept the afternoon away.

18: Up @ 4a because cat vomited in the hall and in the bathroom. Aided by whiskey, wrote a sad letter to Geoffrey likely deflating his own good mood. The senior Jenkners still troublesome re. Didy's treatment. Her mother wants me to send her to quacks in the USA, one of whom injects the patient's own processed urine back into them. Cleaned the house top to bottom. Visa credit card fraud discovered and reported. New card issued.

19: Radiation #4 @ 9:00a. Slept intermittently with gout-ridden foot and ankle. Wrote Nicolas Comeau, then relaxed with Didy and drinks, reviewing the day.

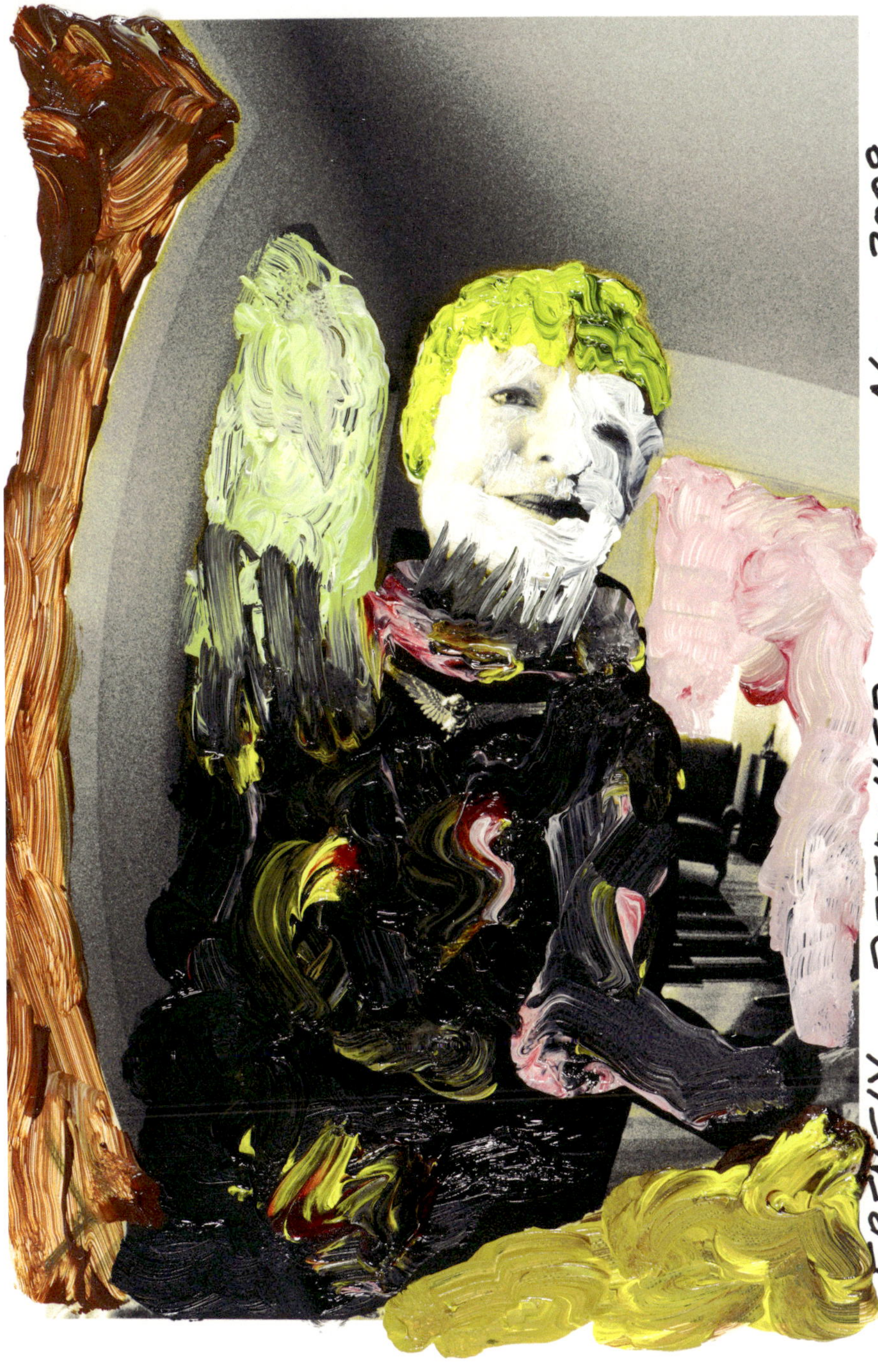

SERENELY DETACHED Nov 2009

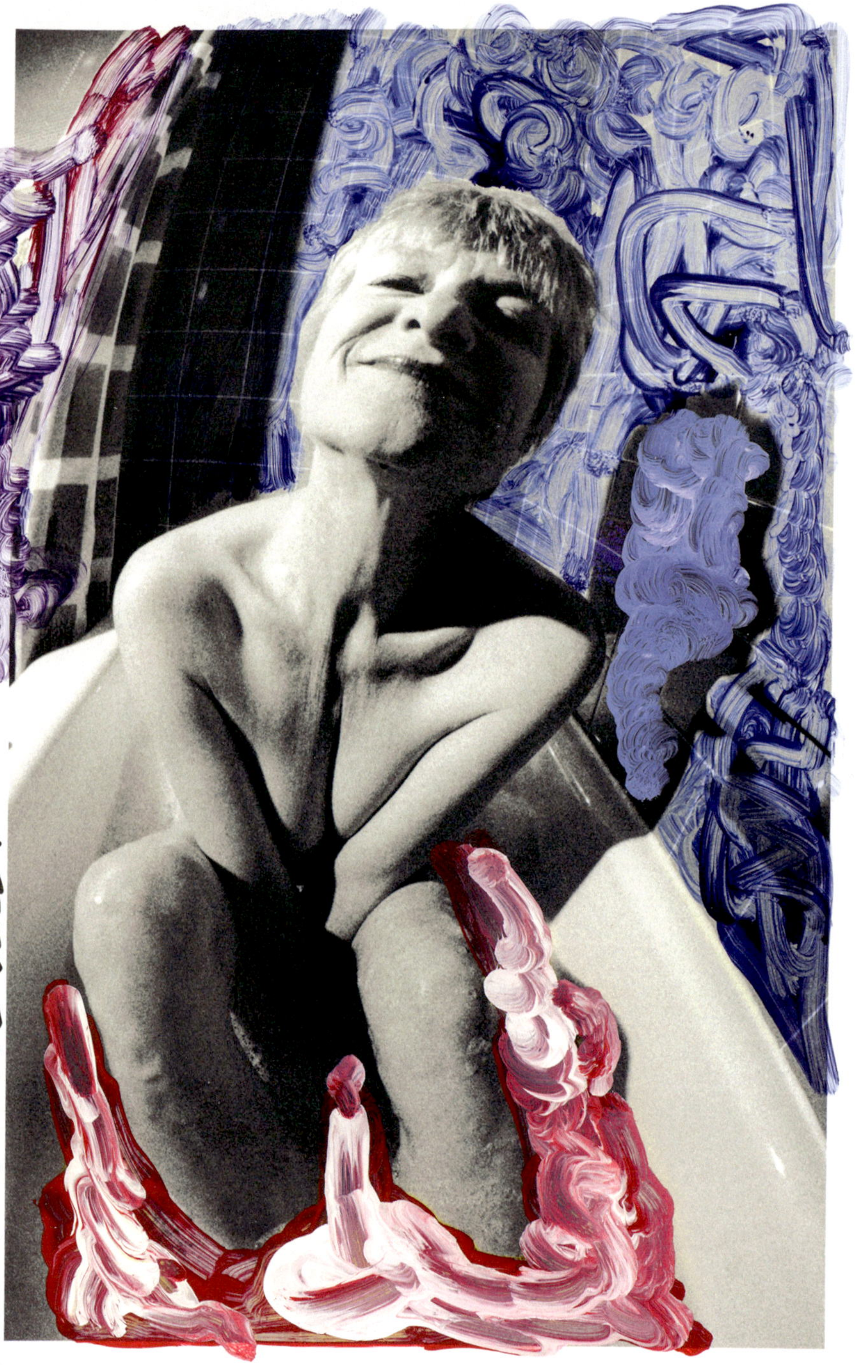

AFTER RADIATION 2009

20: Radiation #5 @ 9:15a then interview with Dr. Maureen Nolan, the radiation oncologist.Long morning at the VG, bad traffic on the way home. Printed Xmas photocards of NSR in the afternoon while Didy slept. In addition to every other fucking thing, I'm upset mightily by the huge fraudulent transactions on my Visa card!

21: Chemo bottle change and radiation #6 @ 11:00a. Lunch at Susanne Swannie's with Mern O'Brien. Quite pleasant considering my troubled past with that woman. Walked our neighbourhood paths among the autumn leaves, then printed photocards while Didy napped.

22: Radiation #7 @ 12:00a. Didy looking very tired this morning even after 12 hours' sleep. A slow and dragging nervous day. Trip to the gallery to pick up files. Feeling diminished.

23: Assembled Xmas cards and envelopes. Then a solid lunch with a bottle of Vouvray. Straightened out Didy's dental insurance claim. Didy fractious and irritable. Radiation #8 @ 4:30p.

24: IJ has severe diarrhea caused by radiation treatments. To pharmacy for medicine. Didy combative and insensitive. She has much to be resentful about. Buried my emotions by gluing photos onto Xmas greeting cards.

25: Heavy tropical storm, violent winds and heavy rain. Tortured sleep with half awake dreams of a terrible future. Didy looking very old before her time. Shot a roll of 35mm on the Widelux at the Prince's Lodge circular music room.

26: Radiation #9 @ 12:15p. Didy suffering and confrontational. Lovely autumn day, but atmosphere in the house is bad. Wrote a poor letter to Geoffrey S.

27: Radiation #10 @ 8:30 a and GP Dr. Somers @ 3:45p. Another bad night of horrible dreams. Didy not really herself. I catch her staring at the floor for minutes at a time. Phoned friends while IJ was at the gallery polishing up the CC grant application.

28: Didy struggled to fuck this morning with chemo bottle and PICC line. She yelped when my cock went into her. Then the run to the hospital for radiation #11 @ 11:00a Exhausting. Applied the annual coat of green Pentox to the deck in the sunny crisp afternoon.

29: Radiation #12 @ 7:30a after an exceptionally bad night. Didy is in pain, her bowels very active and haemorrhoids painful. Shopped while Didy worked on gallery's CC grant. Didy seems indifferent and cold—only her own interests have any significance. I am unhappy. Washed the Rust Check off the VW wagon.

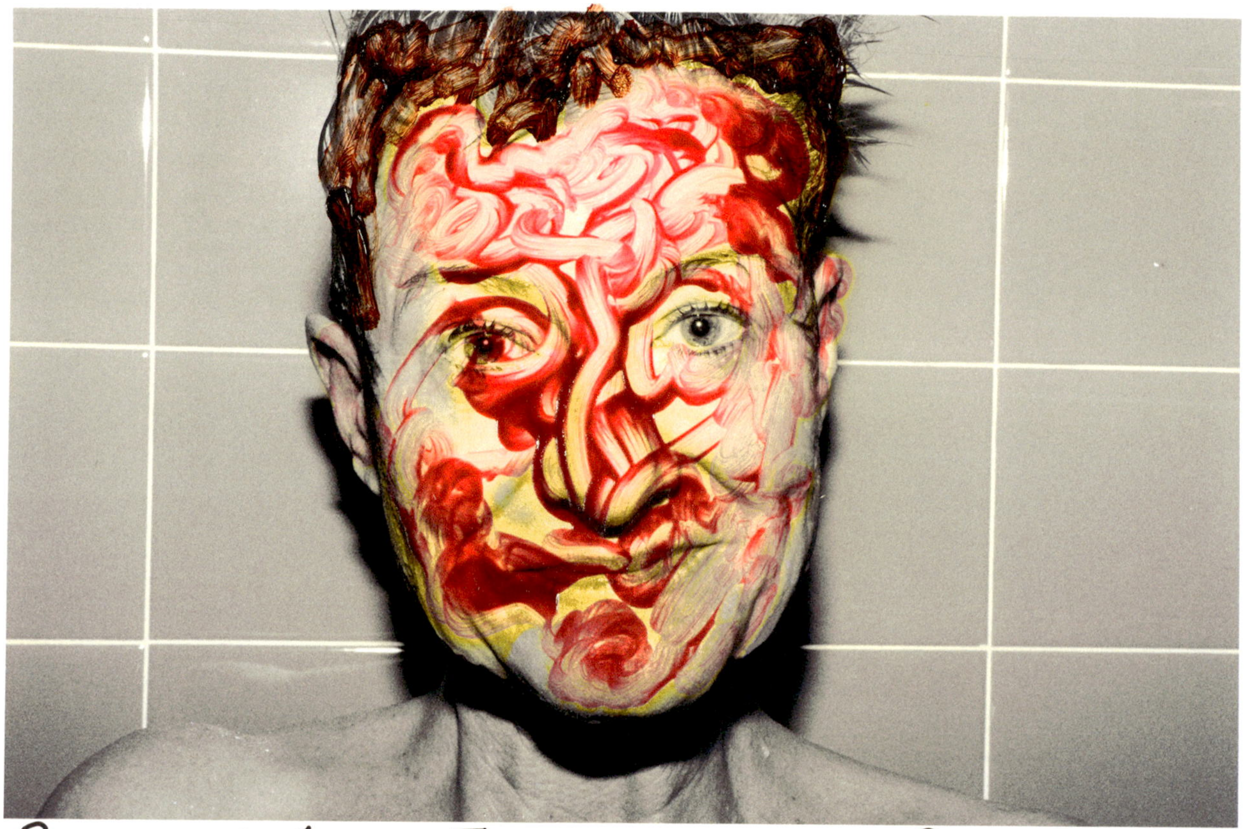

RADIATION & CHEMO EXHAUSTION DEC 2009

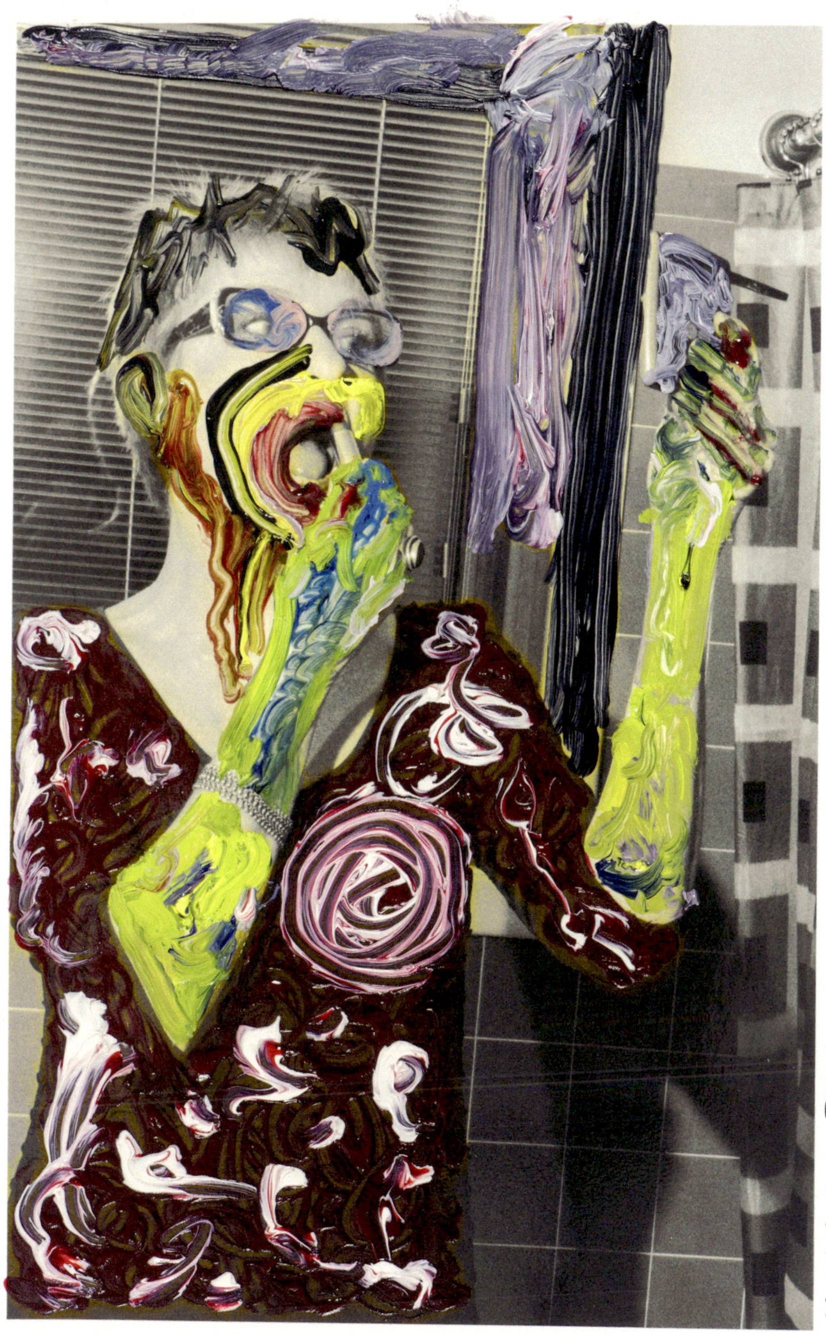

XMAS PARTY 2009

30: Radiation #13 @ 2:25p. Steve Higgins, Jan Peacock, and Micah Lexier visited here. Well meaning, I suppose, but not helpful—stayed far too long and Micah stepped in the cat's water bowl. Fraudulent Visa charges have been removed.

31: Saturday & Halloween. Up early and shopped locally, done by 10a. Moved Mickey's ceramic sculptures from the backyard into the furnace room for the winter. Played Verdi's *Don Carlo* on CD while the wind blew the leaves down the street. Did not go to Pete's and ate leftovers. IJ quite nasty by end of day, in an intentionally hurtful way.

NOVEMBER 2009

1: Up early and alone, cleaned up the kitchen, and wrote a letter to Martha Langford and Donigan Cumming. Didy in foul mood. Says that her cunt is radiation burned. Better than usual joint shopping and afternoon walk. Cooked prime-rib roast beef dinner.

2: Radiation #14 @ 7:45a. Didy not very affectionate and showing more signs of radiation side effects. Met with Donna Grant, licenced practical nurse and cancer treatment coordinator @ 9:45a. Surgery likely in January.

3: Radiation #15 @ 9:30a then a meeting with Dr. Nolan at 10:00a who is pleased with the tumour s shrinkage. The grind continues. Spotted Don Reider, Valerie Dean' supercilious husband at the VG, who looked terrible. Mall shopping with Didy on way home from Cancer Centre. Worked on the Xmas mailout. Cooked tasty nutritious supper.

4: Garon and Marg Awalt for coffee @ 10:00a. Garon very taken with Didy. Very pleasant morning, made our day really. Chemo bottle change @ 1:00p then radiation #16 @ 1:30p.

5: Lunch at the Wooden Monkey with Marjorie Simmins and Silver Donald Cameron. Marjorie a bundle of emotional energy. The Radiation #17 @ 2:45p. With so little reserves of calm any upset is unnerving, even the pleasant ones.

6: Radiation #18 @ 11:15a.First snow. Early morning letter to Geoffrey. Phone message from DTC (Donigan) not responded to. Difficult day, Didy suffering & unpleasant.

7: Slept first part of night downstairs because I was angry with Didy, but back into bed with her @ 2:00a. Minor cock fondling. Wore cotton tights shopping, swollen cock on public display. *Tannhäuser* from the Met in the afternoon. Extensive cooking for today and tomorrow.

8: Didy tried to take my cock inside her but not even the head could get past her burned labia. Vagina is quite possibly contracted as well. Fran and John for lunch. Worked basically all day long cooking and cleaning.

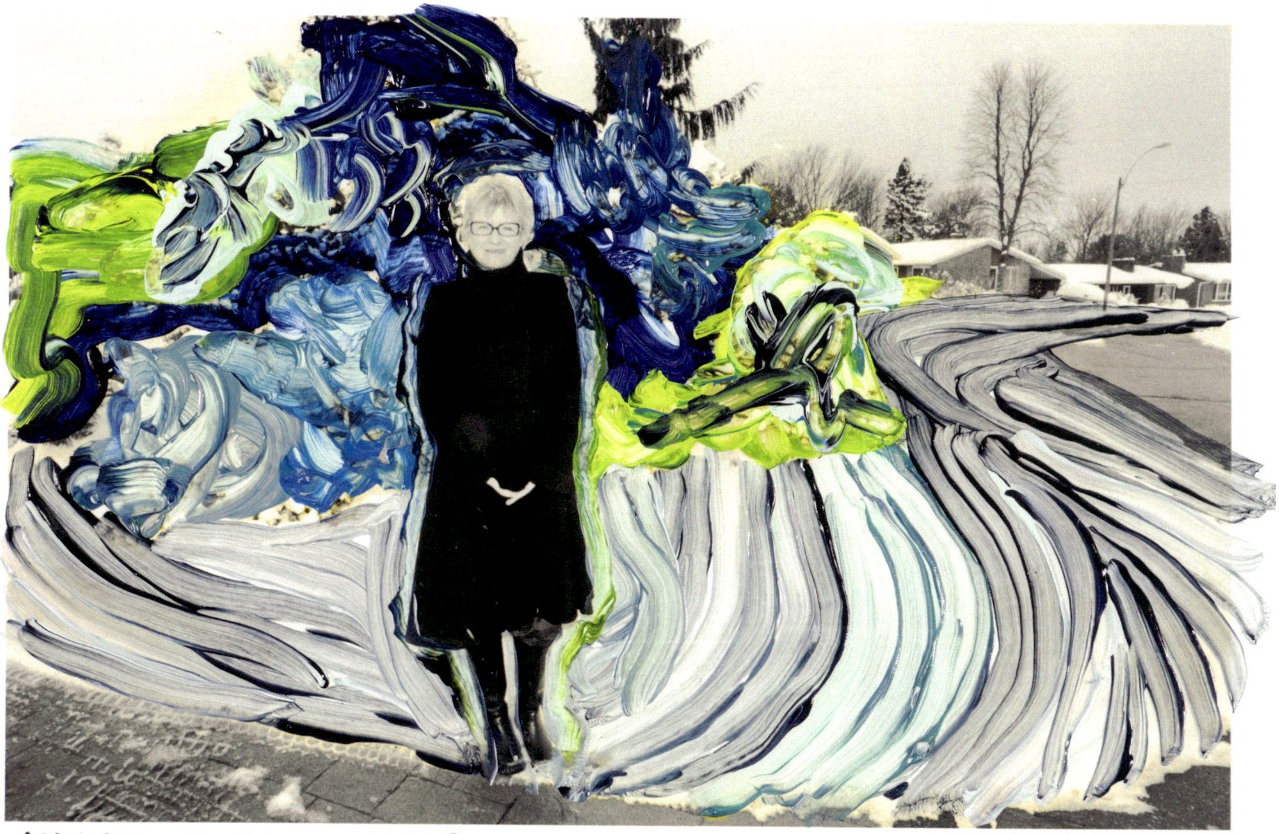

XMAS DAY 2009

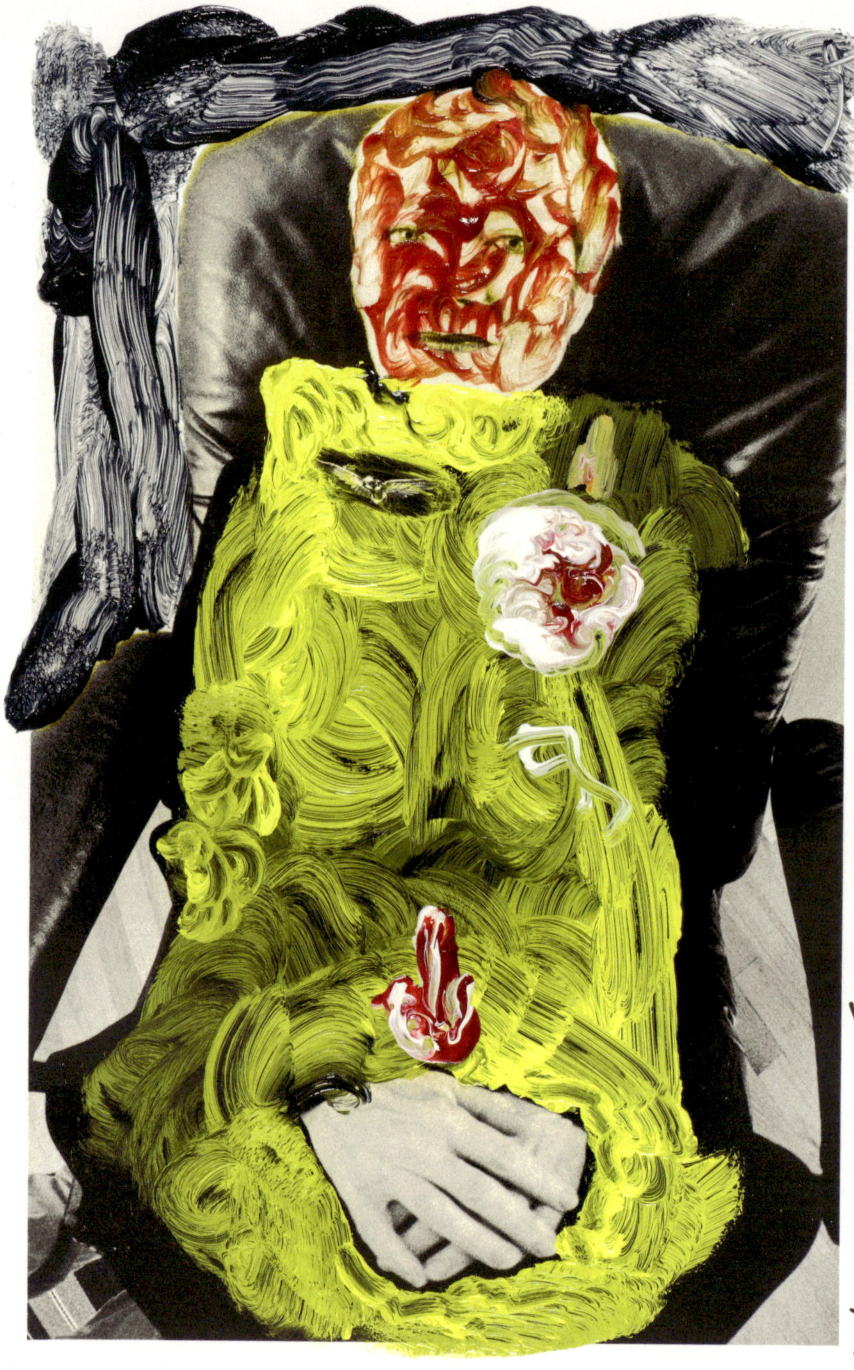

WAITING FOR SURGERY XMAS 2009

9: Radiation #19 @ 7:15a. Didy very bothered by her mother's aggression re. the standard of care she's receiving in Halifax. E-mail exchange with IJ's sister Karin about the progress of Didy's treatment. The shocking news is that Karin's Wally has prostate cancer and is scheduled for surgery very soon.

10: Chemo bottle change @ 10a then Radiation #20 @ 10:30a. Much conversation with IJ re. Wally's cancer diagnosis and her crazy mother's ballistic phone calls. Very tired of that. Appalled by life's outcomes.

11: Armistice Day. A day of rest from the hell of the cancer treatment regime. My thoughts very much in the past. Life has deteriorated since retirement, as I knew it would. Mere survival now.

12: Radiation #21 @ 2:45p. Another long day of not being myself, doing things that I don't want to do. How terrible life has turned out to be. Is there any way out of this trap? Must endure while waiting for events to save me.

13: Friday the 13th, Radiation #22 @ 1:45p. Quiet morning at home. Selected recipients of the worst Xmas photocard—LFH sucking on a catheter inserted into my semi-erect penis. Apparently Alexa McDonough will call at the house with IJ's ironclad letter.

14: Very difficult night for Didy, severe diarrhea and cramps, had to take Imodium medication. But she slept late, 8:30a, and woke in good spirits. Shopped at Pete's for food and ran into NSCAD's infamous 'Woman from Minnesota', Susan Mac.

15: Starved for sex this morning, a grand teasing blow job would have been welcome. Some penis fondling did take place. Tired of living in a dirty house and doing chores without end. Fran and John for lunch.

16: Radiation #23 @ 12:15p. A 'Death in Venice' moment when I recalled ogling a small-titted beauty at the Crystall & Luckett wine store on Saturday last.

17: Chemo bottle and PICC line removal @ 10a, radiation #24 @ 10:30p, then Didy to dentist, Russell Mac Sween @ 12:20p. A fine autumn day to have Didy freed at last from the chemo bottle. The stay at the VG Cancer Centre this morning was so long. Drinks all afternoon, e-mail from NSR.

18: Last radiation treatment #25 @ 12:15p on another fine day. To postoffice for more stamps then food shopping. Made very nice dinner with Australian red champagne. IJ suffering from side effects and not with much grace.

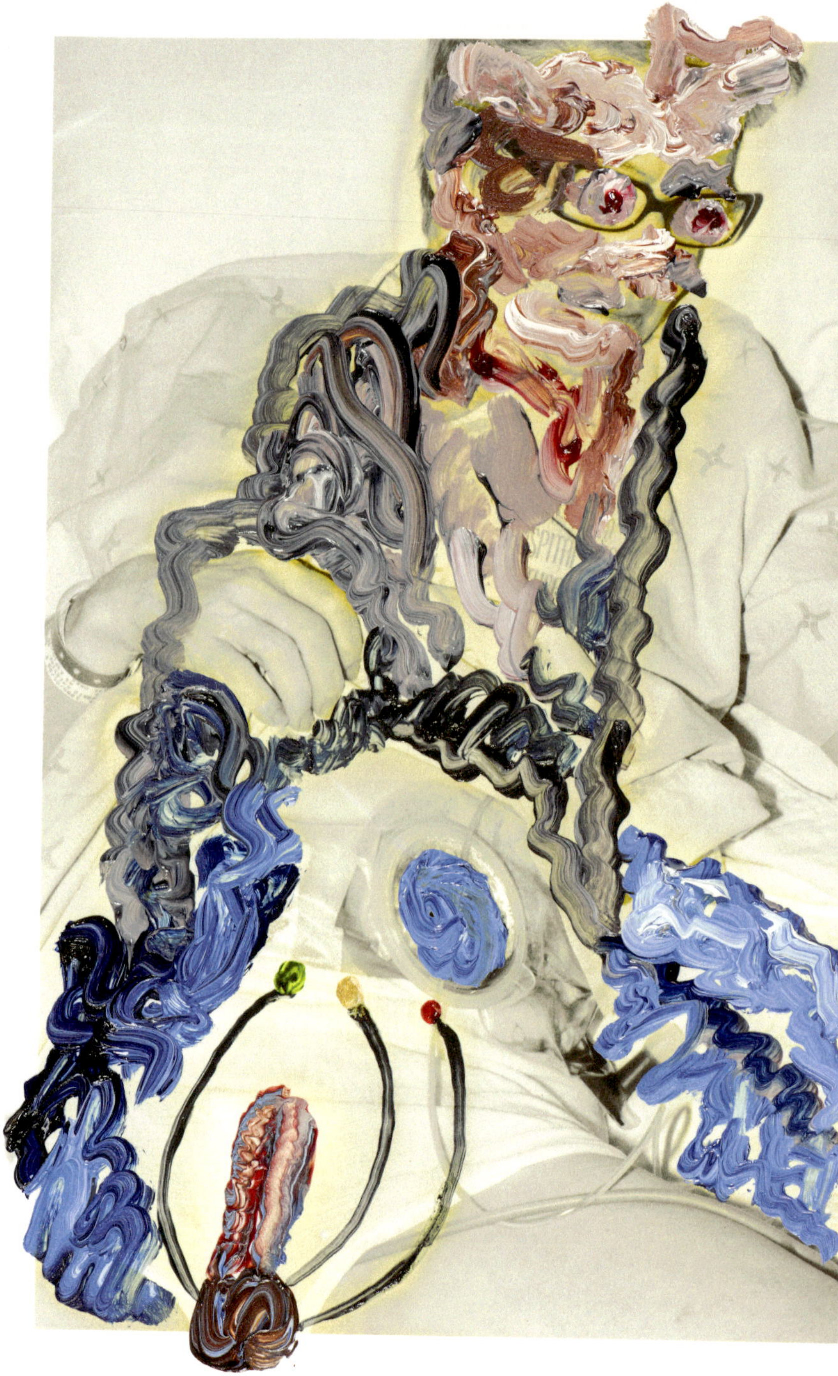

EXCISION ACCOMPLISHED 15 JAN 2010

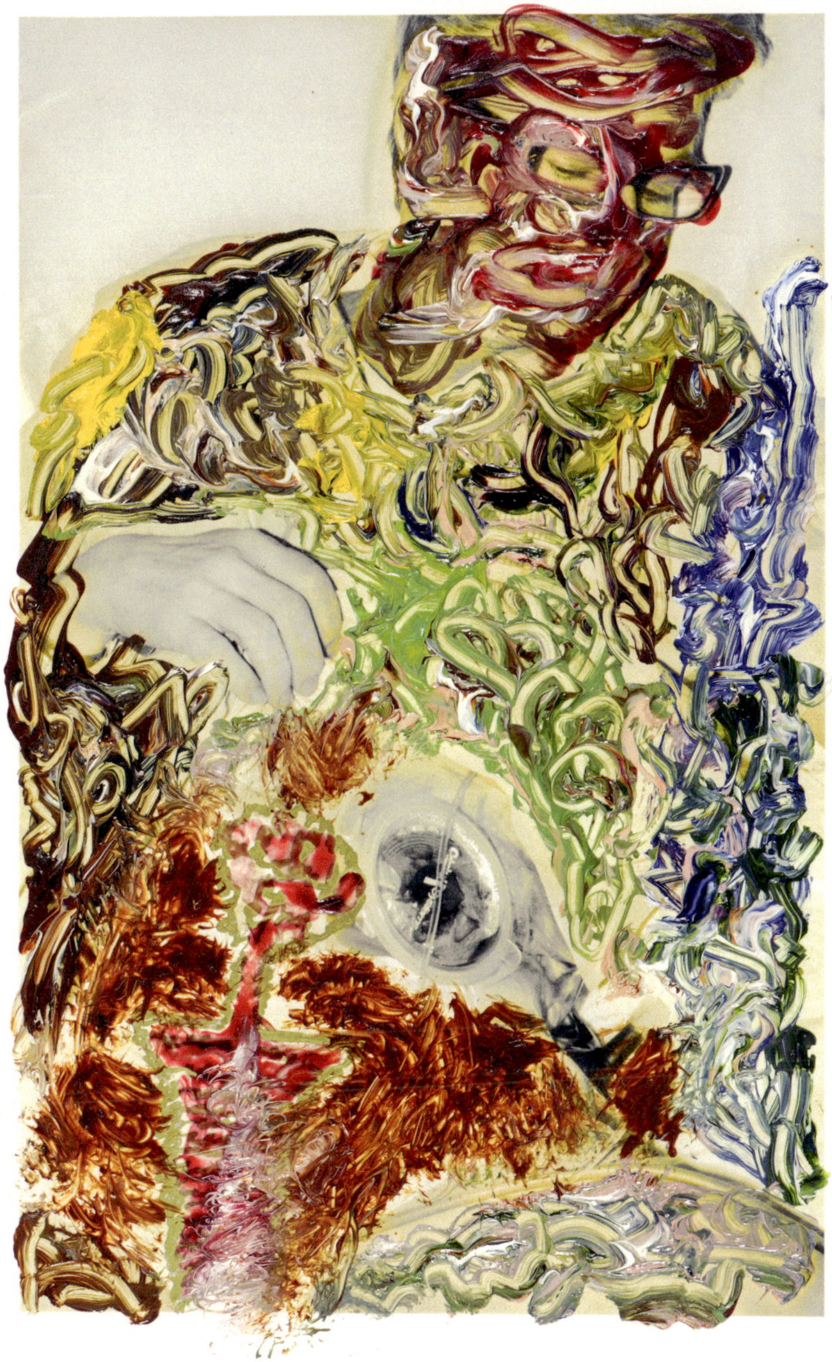

EXCISION ACCOMPLISHED 15 JAN 2010

19: Arose @ 4a as Didy was too restless to sleep with. Wrote 5 short letters on a glass of whiskey. Another beautiful day.

20: Sexual frustration and IJ's ingratitude the dominant theme here. Only spiritual growth will save me now. The monstrous mother has had an accident, a fall of some sort, perhaps it will shut her up. Didy adversarial, I slept downstairs in terrible pain, likely passing kidney stones.

21: Up @ 4a to write a response to Geoffrey's bleak letter on his family's troubles. Wolfgang phoned early re. 'Mum's' condition, a bit more serious than first reported. Just one more aspect of things around here being all about Jenkners.

22: Fifth anniversary of the death of IJ's former partner Mickey Handy. In need of down and dirty sex. Solid letters to Chester Pelkey and Martha. IJ shouted, "The house is really dirty. When are you going to clean it?" It's easy to see where this is going. Didy approached the subject of joint suicide after observing how old she looked in the bathroom mirror. It's all just loose talk on her part, but I have been to the edge on that one.

23: Much too much to-do about IJ's lunatic mother. Long walk to the post office to mail letter to Martha re. Oxford University Press book, *The Visual Arts in Canada* with permission to publish *Hands Clasped, 40th birthday*, 1983, from *The Pictures of Ellen*.

24: Slept better than usual, as did Didy. Living together all day every day is excessively revealing. Selfish and inconsiderate to the core and protected from any consequences by enormous insensitivity. That's merely what I see. Didy is going through hell: cancer, the recent late in life marriage, and her parents crumbling.

25: Printed the last batch of Xmas photocards, title "Micturition on Detractors." Didy had an hour or so of being her old wonderful self. Walked together to Sobeys, that tired her out completely.

26: Up well before 4a to work on Xmas mailout and e-mail to Donigan. Communications with Martha re. OUP book. Completed Xmas cards. Very angry with Didy re. indifference.

27: IJ's sister Karin's birthday. Didy 'lunching' with idiot Prof. Randi in the middle of the afternoon. Cleaned the house meanwhile. Hate living this way, a servant to Didy and the cat. I must be, I have to be, more merciful and magnanimous. The apprehension of the surgery weighs heavily on us both.

28: Didy at her most aggravating, wilfully so. She let the cat in the negative cabinet while my back was turned. Disrespectful and contrary at every step. Then too drunk to make any sense. I write this, but hopefully don't show it.

29: Slept downstairs the entire night, as usual Didy awoke with no apparent knowledge of her hurtful behaviour. Lovely late autumn day, bright and windy. Cooked extensive Sunday dinner. Sexually frustrated.

30: Kept waiting while IJ blabbed on the phone to her girl pal Gina. Mailed print to Khalia Scott in Ottawa for photo-school benefit print sale. Very short tempered. Didy's radiation burns much improved. She even raised the matter of fucking.

DECEMBER 2009

1: Didy is reawakening sexually and much more affectionate. Placed Light Impressions order. Sexual intercourse with Didy that was somewhat painful for her. Overseas mailout ready.

2: Appointment with surgeon Dr. Jamieson @ 10a, VG 9th floor GI unit. Operation is called,"Abdominal Peritoneal Resection," resulting in a "Total Mesorectal Excision." Translation: surgical removal of anus, rectum, descending colon, and lymph nodes; accomplished by incisions in front and back, in front from navel to pubic bone and in back from pelvis down to the peritoneum. The removals will result in some displacement of remaining organs. Surgery tentatively scheduled for 7th of January.

3: Cold rain filled day but warm and cunty inside with Didy, who is almost feeling OK. Not for long though, Didy on the phone with her loser pal Morgan Wood the indigenous indigent.

4: Don't want to live this way. Death is so attractive. Let them, the women, sort it out. A bleak day, women are so cruel. Ah! To be out of here, with one shotgun round, so near, near. I will abide with the backyard dog's grave alone.

5: Opera *Der Rosenkavalier.* Memorial service at NSCAD Port Campus for Jerry Ferguson @ 3p. A very moving ceremony, the aged art historian, Dennis Young, friend and colleague of the deceased gave a fervent, wide-ranging, and genuine talk about his friend. The usual art school poseurs attended. Miss Heller was there representing her sister, the painter Susanna Heller. She presented IJ with one of her sister's drawings. IJ not pleased.

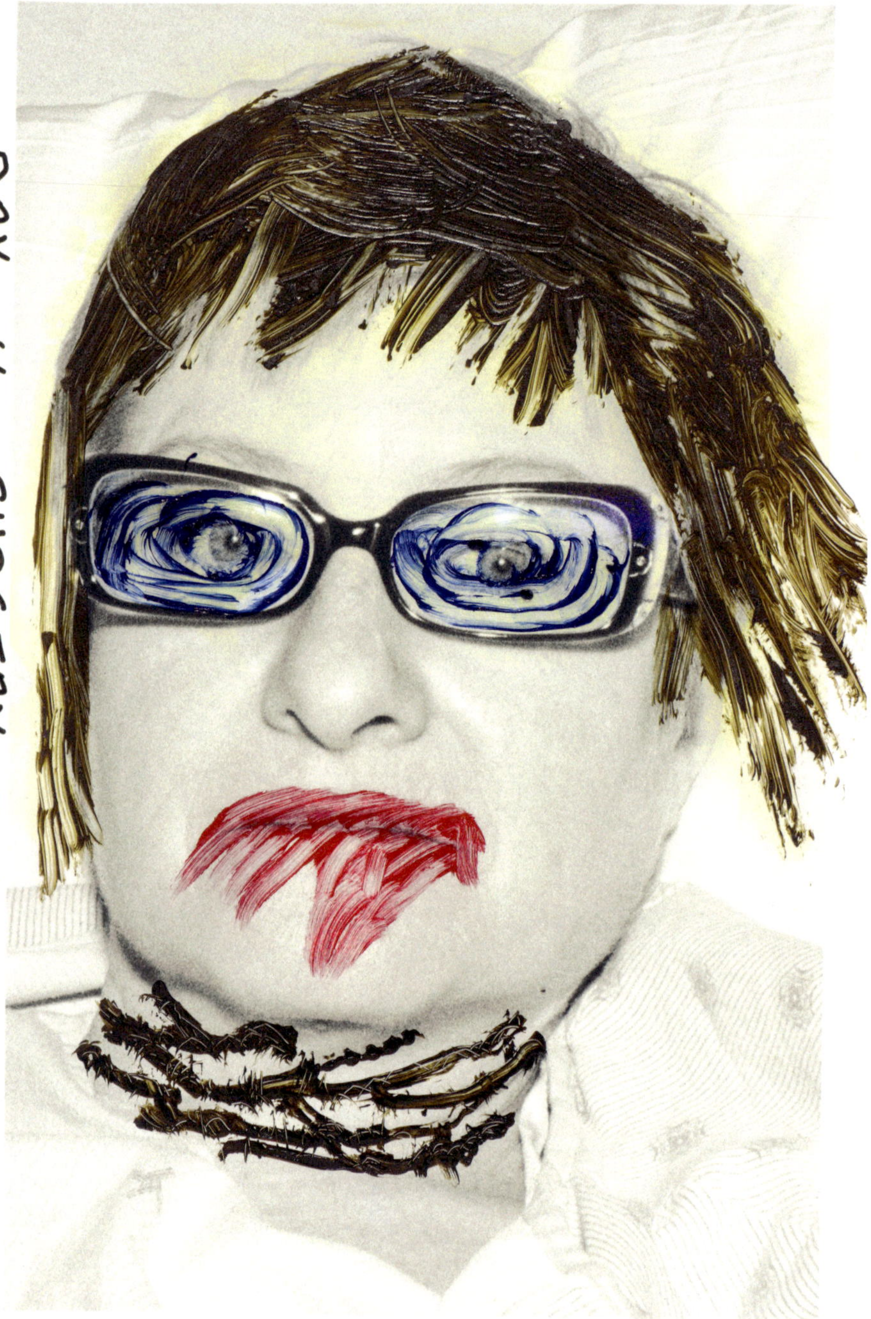

DAY after SURGERY 2010

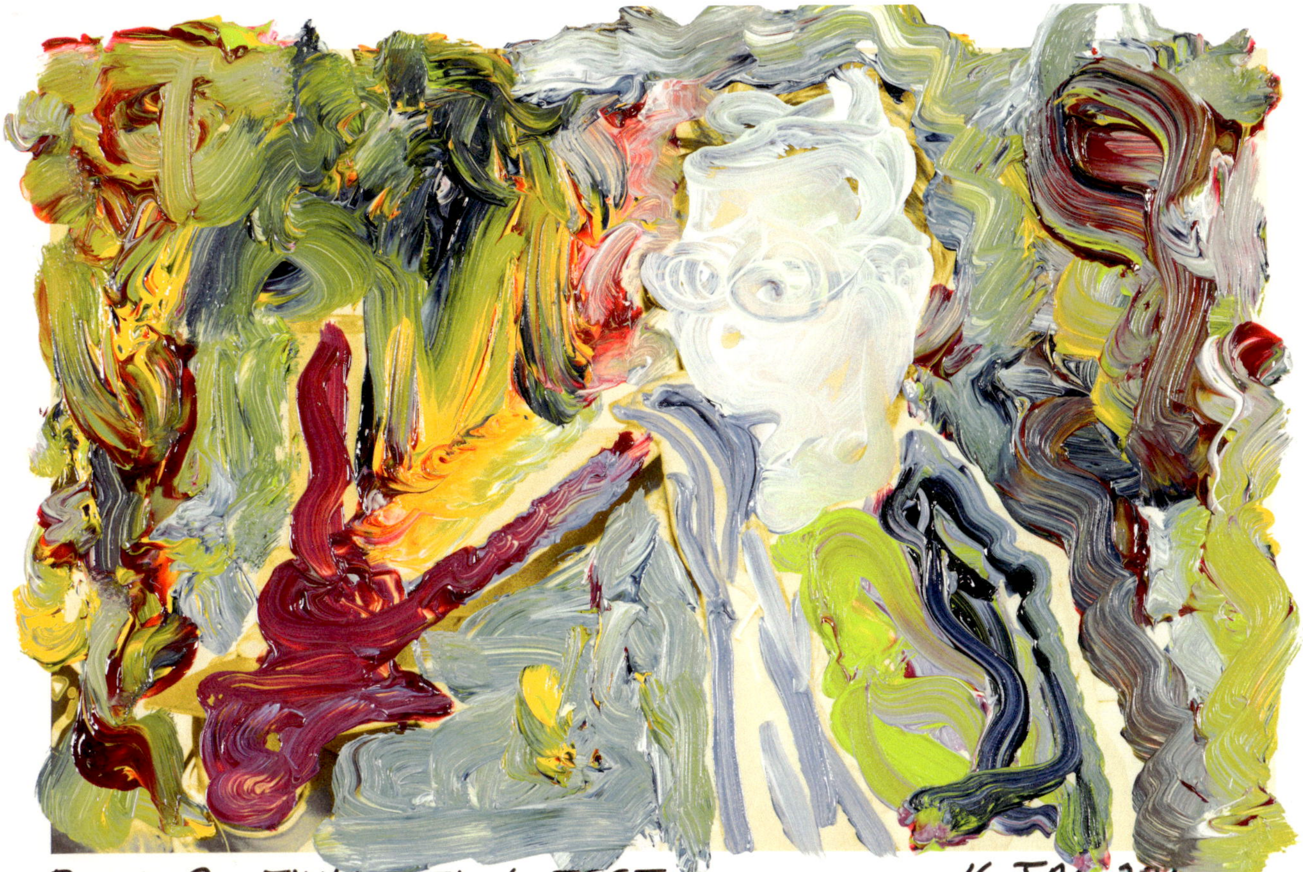

POST-OP EXHALATION TEST 16 JAN 2010

6: Winter Storm. Could not drive to Pete's in Bedford, walked to Sobeys. Surprisingly no Sunday morning phone call from IJ's Elders in Mississauga. Wrote letters during the night to Kahlia Scott and Martha.

7: Juicy sex in the morning. Didy drank whiskey all afternoon, became drunk and combative. Walked away from the red wine she spilled on the floor and ate at the dinner table with her bare hands. Huge fight ensued.

8: Bad nightmares of the screaming out loud kind. Didy serene in the morning, as is her way. A more sensible day, Italian soup and a very German supper.

9: Gallery staff Xmas luncheon at Japanese Mikimoto restaurant. Lithium batteries arrived. No sign of the German baking from Munich though. Cleaned up the bathroom mess Didy left. Enjoyed the luncheon and socializing.

10: Slept mostly downstairs but returned to Didy's bed @ 4a and fucked at dawn. Mailed out domestic Xmas photocards. Received 10 more 2007 MSVU catalogues to replenish stock. Light Impressions charged Visa, but failed to ship any supplies, but I'll adapt.

11: Slept well downstairs. Appointment at the Surgery Clinic @ 1:30p and 2p. Traumatic interview with 'Stoma' nurse. She tattooed the place on IJ's abdomen where the transverse colon will exit (ileostomy), and the ostomy pouch will attach. She explained the mechanics of living with an ileostomy in vivid and excruciating detail. The surgical outcome seems quite unimaginable.

12: Xmas party at the home of Peter Dykhuis and Jayne Wark starting @ 8p. Strange morning with IJ fucking off to her beauty parlour appointment early. House cleaning & meal preparation. Didy wore her fancy red wedding dress to the party, presumably for the last time. It was at last year's party that Peter & Jayne champagne-toasted our wedding in Mississauga, then days away. This year's party was just as grand, and I was more relaxed.

13: Drove home drunk and safely. Woke to a get-down at-home day, no shower. Busy with photo *minutiae*. Put expired flowers on the dog's backyard grave. Didy got very drunk and passed out on the sofa in a mean-spirited mood. Very difficult to get Didy to bed, her being so nasty.

14: As always, no mention of this made in the morning. To Belgian bakery, German deli, and Liquor store. Arrivals of Xmas gifts from NSR and Donigan Cumming. Another boozy day, but no unpleasantness.

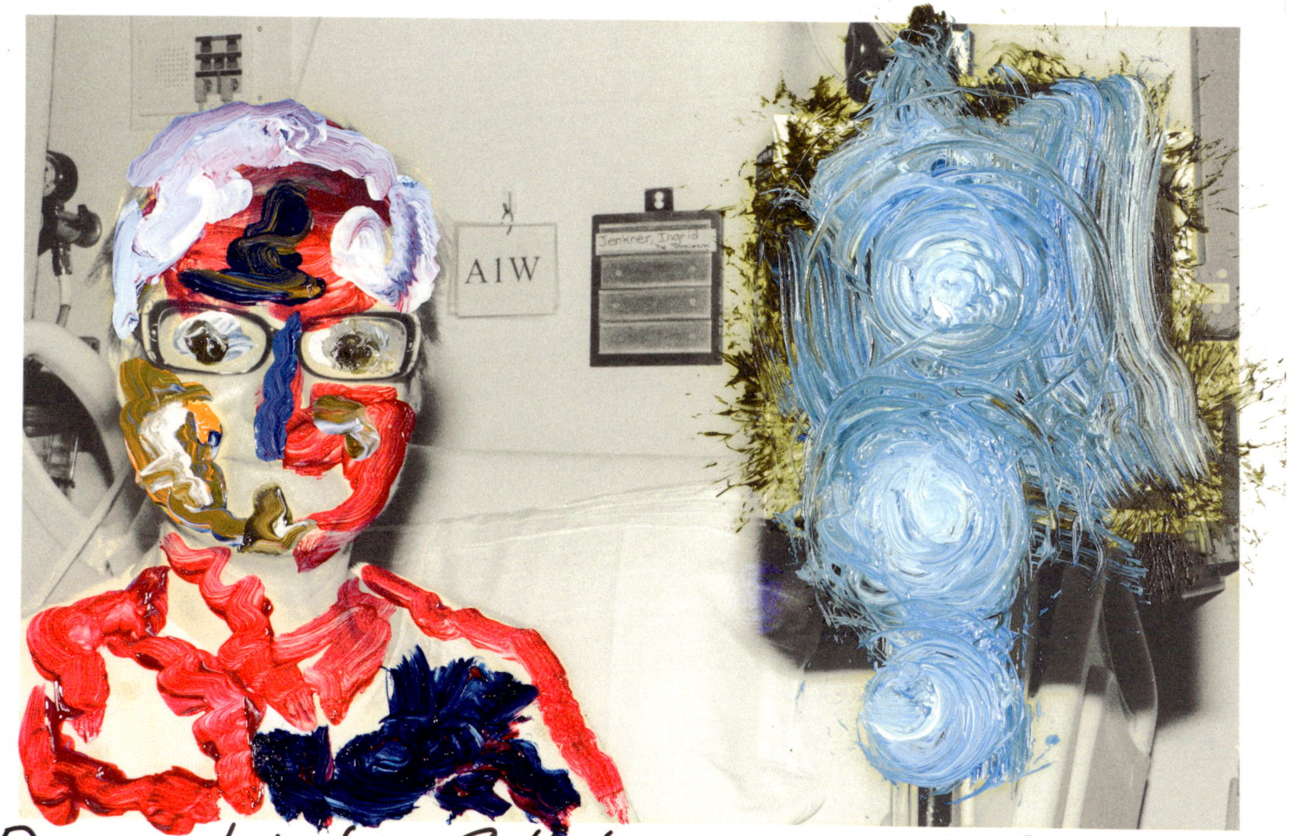

Disconnected from Catheters 18 JAN 2010

15: Up @ 1:30a to write to Donigan, then with a Cialis-assisted erection got back in bed with Didy @ 4a where her tight little cunt was waiting, swollen and wet. Daytime, Didy out of control on whiskey, tearful and afraid of death. Not a pleasant person to be with at the moment. She is the hand that fate dealt me and I'll endure.

16: Slept all night long with Didy and fucked her hard in the morning. Thoroughly vacuumed the house and cooked a good dinner. Xmas cards and other acknowledgements of the mailout coming in now.

17: 1st wife Linda to visit @ 2p. She, according to our long standing custom, brought a Maritime dark fruitcake, my mother's recipe, while I had a Belgian Stollen for her and Peter. Loved talking to the two wives, who genuinely like each other.

18: A very cold and wintry day, and a long and boozy one. Didy did lose it near the end but I was successful in ignoring that. The crippled, one-footed crow, that I've fed for five years died in the backyard.

19: Met broadcast season opened with *Les Contes d'Hoffmann*. Huge shop at Pete's in preparation for the Susanne Swannie lunch tomorrow. Cooked supper @ 3p to avoid Didy passing out. Opera was excellent. Martha happy with her 56th birthday flowers.

20: The Susanne Swannie lunch went well with Peggy MacKinnon unexpectedly joining us. Afternoon was pleasant with fireplace going and music playing while a severe winter storm raged outside. Phone message from NSR.

21: Winter Solstice. An enjoyable lazy day. Much snow shovelling and meal preparation (full roast beef dinner). Disingenuous Xmas card from perfidious Martha Hanna. She's on her way out the door of the Canadian Museum of Contemporary Photography, destroyed by the Harper government. A better director than Hanna might have saved it.

22: Sex @ 4a then off to the hospital. Pre-op exam at the Victoria General @ 10:30a 10th floor, lasted 3 hours. Another reality-inducing day at the VG. IJ's tumours have shrunk enormously under the 25 radiation treatments plus the 24/7 chemo and are ready for the surgical removal. Homeward to recover with whiskey and the longed for Xmas mail.

23: 1st wedding anniversary. I go to Dr. Russell MacSween for extensive dental work, porcelain crown. A couple of drinks then comestibles shopping for the holidays. Surprise personal visit from the university president, Alexa McDonough, with the letter for IJ and flowers.

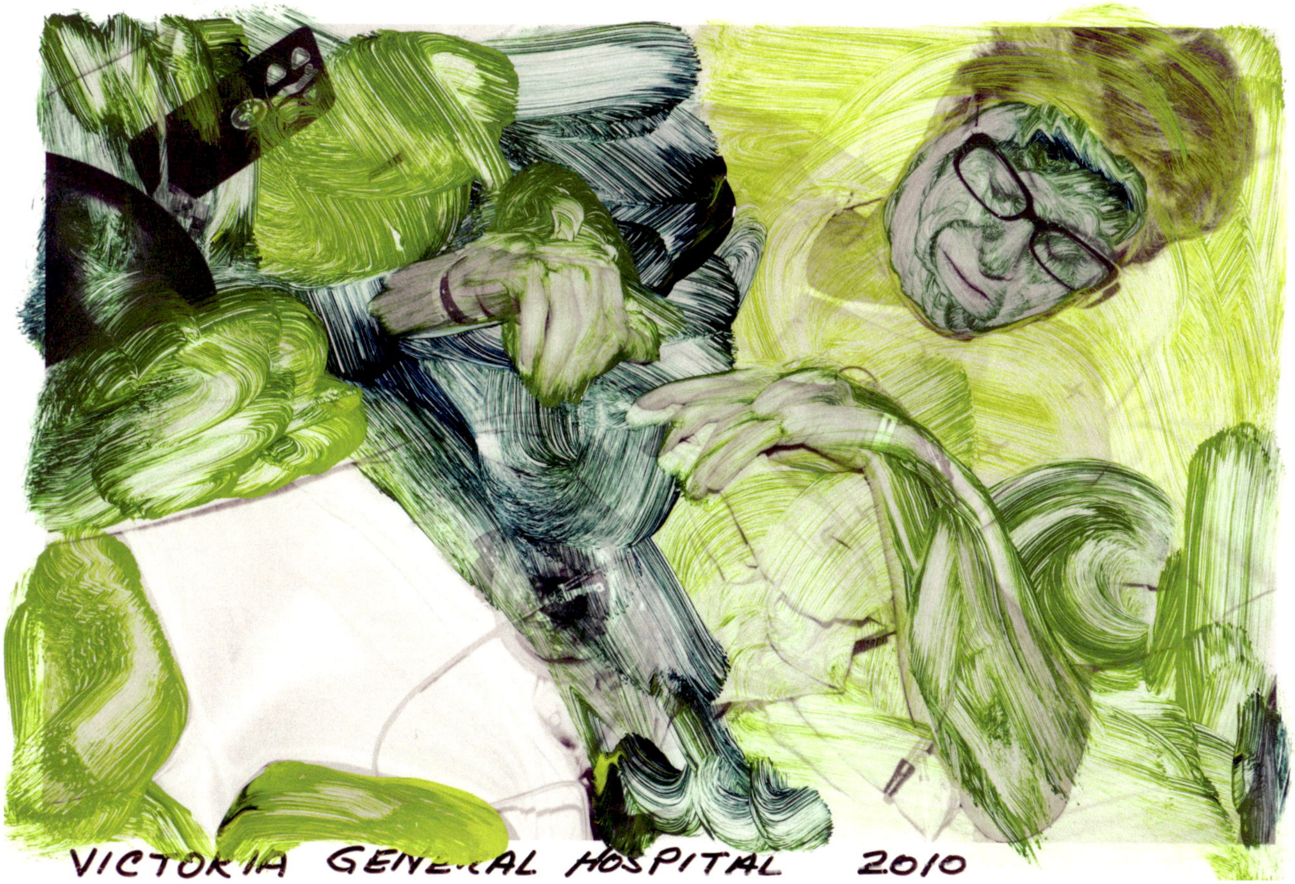

VICTORIA GENERAL HOSPITAL 2010

24: Christmas Eve day. Invited for dinner at Armshore Drive, Marjorie Simmins & Silver Donald Cameron. Fucked vigorously @ 6a and then again @ 3p. Lots of incoming Xmas cards. Print sale at Ottawa's School of the Photographic Arts exceeded expectations. Didy fractious and happy. Nice time with Marjorie & SDC, the mood upbeat and sensible. Home and dry.

25: Christmas Day. Talked at length with Wolfgang who is not a chatty type. Dinner at Fran & John's, I helped rescue the undercooked free-range turkey and used surgical skills to carve it for the guests

26: Boxing Day. Opera *Electra*. Long conversation with Martha Langford & Donigan Cumming then lunch and a fire with an ambitious afternoon fuck on the livingroom sofa. Shot Didy post-coital in a bubble bath.

27: More balls-deep sex during the night. Didy in a good mental space, until she spent all afternoon on the bottle & acted badly by suppertime.

28: Lubricious sex @ dawn. Didy worried and fretful about surgery and its consequences. I ordered personalized stationary from Crane & Co. Also a black camera bag from B+H. Didy sullen and mean. What a 1st year of a marriage this has been. Gloss worn with the worst yet to come. IJ seems not to care, wilful and uncaring.

29: VW wagon has exhaust system problem. To bakery for 'Hearth' bread. Didy very worried about her life expectancy. Wonderful Xmas cards from S&C and Nicolas Comeau. Solidly fatherly phone call from Wolfgang.

30: Very cold & bright. Didy very distressed—trying to be good to her. Enjoyed shopping & lunching at Pete's. Lovely big bouquet of flowers sent by Chester Pelkey, who could ill afford such an extravagance.

31: New Year's Eve 2009. Warranty repair to 2004 VW Jetta. Xmas card with poem intended I think for Astrid but sent to Tangmere from George Elliott Clarke. Oxford University Press editors want to use *Clasped Hands* on back cover of book (later squashed by the publisher).

JANUARY 2010

1: Up extra early to e-mail Martha and Miss Heller. Both responded in unsatisfactory ways. IJ drank all day & I had to put her to bed without supper. Who wants to cook for a sloppy drunk?

2: Opera *Hänsel und Gretel.* E-mail from Martha, justifiably bitter about the demise of the CMCP. "The Canadian Gov't wasted ten years of my life." But she's pleased about the back cover of the OUP book. Fierce winter storm. Didy's drinking is controlled. Opera and heavy snow, thoughts of Richard Simmins, now dead ten years, at pre-Christmas 1999.

3: Heavy snow shovelling, my back close to an attack. Elders called Didy at length. No shower today. Prolonged quality sex. "I love the way you fuck me." Drank slowly all day. The dread of the upcoming surgery on the 7th ever-present and intensifying.

4: Large box of beautifully packaged German Christmas baking finally arrived from Munich. A day of light whiskeys and video. Didy difficult to handle, obnoxious, self-absorbed, selfish, and inconsiderate.

5: Operation day looms. Delivered German Christmas Stollen around the town. Made lunch and then an early supper, trying to keep Didy from despair and drunkenness. "We got married too late in life." Watched video *Rumpole of the Bailey* to kill time.

6: Day before surgery. Two letters from Geoffrey in Calgary. Tense and edgy day. Didy did not have a drink and neither did I until late in the day. Many phone calls from well wishers. Made preparations to communicate with the Elders post-op—I will phone Wolfgang, and not the crazy mother, @ 10a each day.

7: Operation day. At Victoria General @ 6:45a. Didy prepped and in the OR anteroom by 9:15a. Waited there for 6 hours, as emergency cases repeatedly preempted IJ's surgery. At 3:00p the operation was cancelled and rescheduled a week hence on the 14th. With elation we motored home through a snow storm for comfort food and large whiskeys.

8: Recovery day, both of us utterly exhausted. Placed Chester's flowers on the dog's backyard grave. Whiskey for lunch with cheese and Linda's German fruitcake. Calm and thoughtful today. I don't want Didy's beautiful body carved up.

9: Opera *Der Rosenkavalier.* Another sad and happy day. Did not go to the Belgian bakery as usual, saturated with Valium and self-pity. But that passed and we sallied forth to Pete's and the wine shop. Saw the exquisite, diminutive, vivacious, East Indian cashier. Didy drank too much and didn't eat much supper. Poor sweet thing.

10: A long 14-hours in bed with two sustained intervals of sexual intercourse. Healing the Didy with my cock and cum. Today a calmer matter. Reading and thoughtfulness. Interrupted by Didy getting drunk and offensive. Slept downstairs.

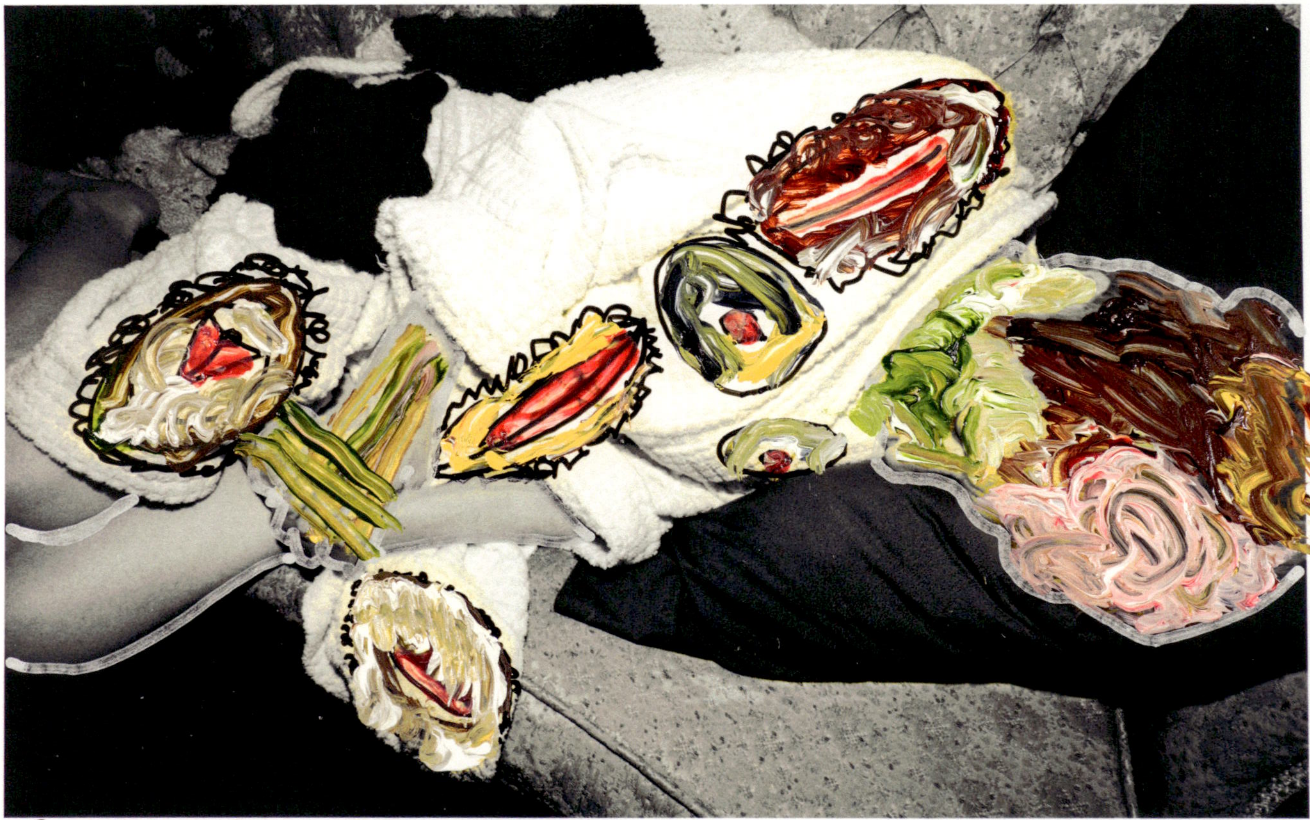

RECOVERING FROM SURGERY JANUARY 2010

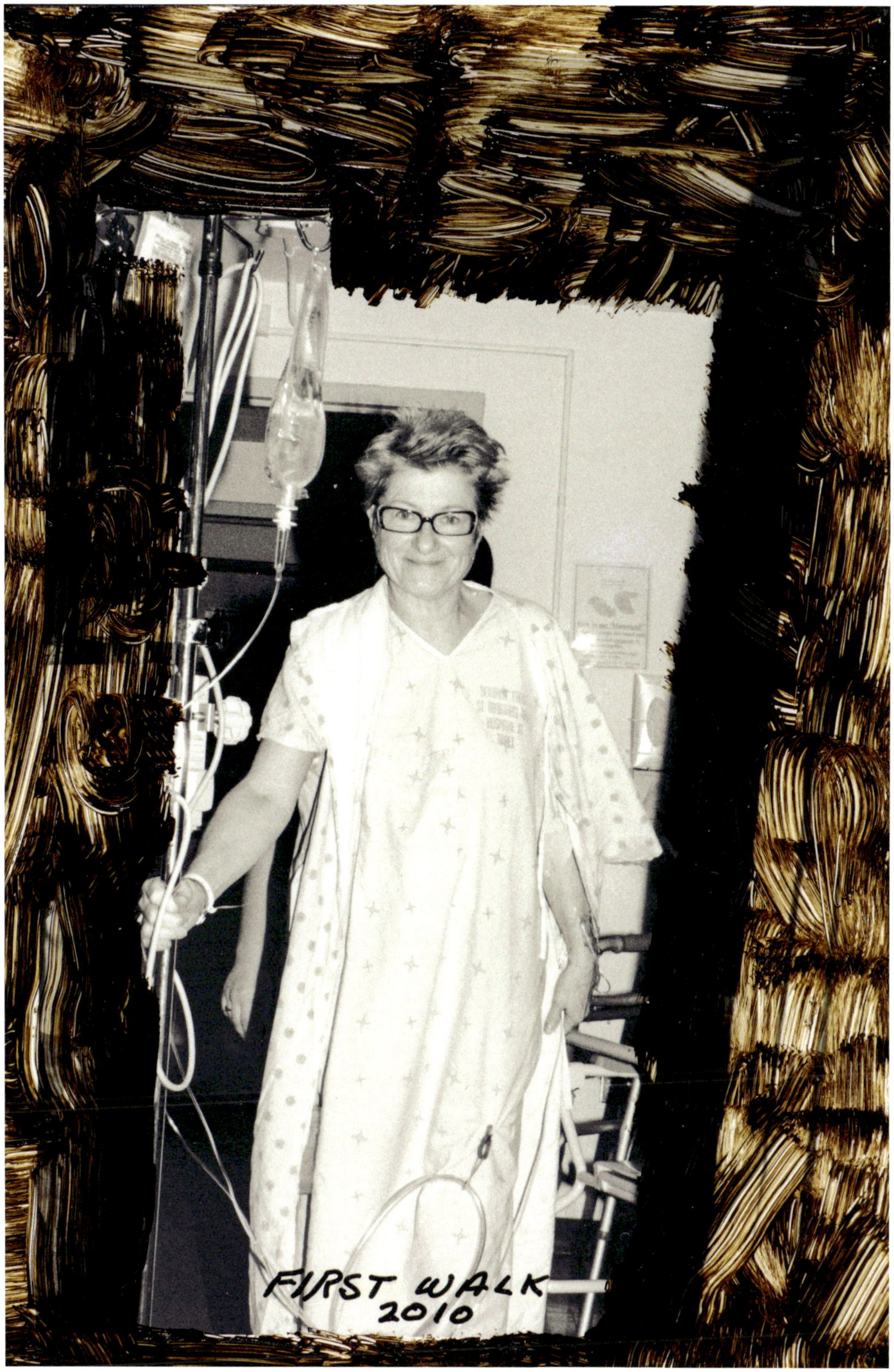
FIRST WALK
2010

11: Extremely cold and clear. Made soup in the morning as a fence mending exercise. Didy slightly contrite and less nervous. No showers or dressing. Didy awfully tired and obviously worried.

12: Not sleeping at all well, switching between beds and then up @ 4a. Some house cleaning and laundry. Lunch out at the Brooklyn Warehouse, then retrieved VW Jetta with new oxygen sensor. Pleading e-mail from Miss Heller.

13: Up early after sleeping well for a change. E-mails to NSR & LFH. A calmer day before surgery than last week. A strange day with stupid people phoning. Made last shots of IJ before disfigurement tomorrow.

14: Operation Day (& Linda's 65th birthday). At the Victoria General @ 8:45a, endless waiting, in the OR waiting room by 11:45a, then more emergencies delayed matters. Didy wheeled in @ 3p. Numb with anxiety and physically & mentally exhausted, I repaired to the dingy and dilapidated waiting rooms reserved for relatives. Gradually the place thinned out until I was the only one remaining. Then sometime after 6p, Dr. Jamieson came in the room and sat with me in his operating room attire. Instead of his gruff self-protective manner, he was kindly and understanding, but still clinical. All had gone well, he said, and enumerated all the body parts he had excised. Drove home in a snow storm and called Wolfgang. Two whiskeys and went to bed.

15: Slept fitfully and up early to send a broadcast e-mail to those waiting for news. Bad nerves and mounting anxiety. Didy courageous and determined, though a pitiful sight to behold. Photographed her in her hospital bed with her wounds on full display. God help us.

16: Opera, the unlovely *Carmen*. So quiet and lovely here with Bulger the cat. Shopped for comestibles then to the hospital. Didy not so alert or energetic as she was yesterday. Photographed a technician installing a catheter in IJ's back for continuous opiate delivery. The pain killing meds have been adjusted upward making her very drowsy. Spoke to Wolfgang and Peggy Mac.

17: Cleaned the house thoroughly before going to the hospital. Didy sleepy and groggy and vomiting into a basin. Washed her hair for her in the patient's bathroom dragging along the heavy duty IV pole with its tubes and peristaltic pump. We haltingly talked, neither of us ourselves to ourselves. Then home to cook a 'Sunday dinner' of sardines on toast. Lots of phone messages that went begging. Took a Valium and collapsed in bed.

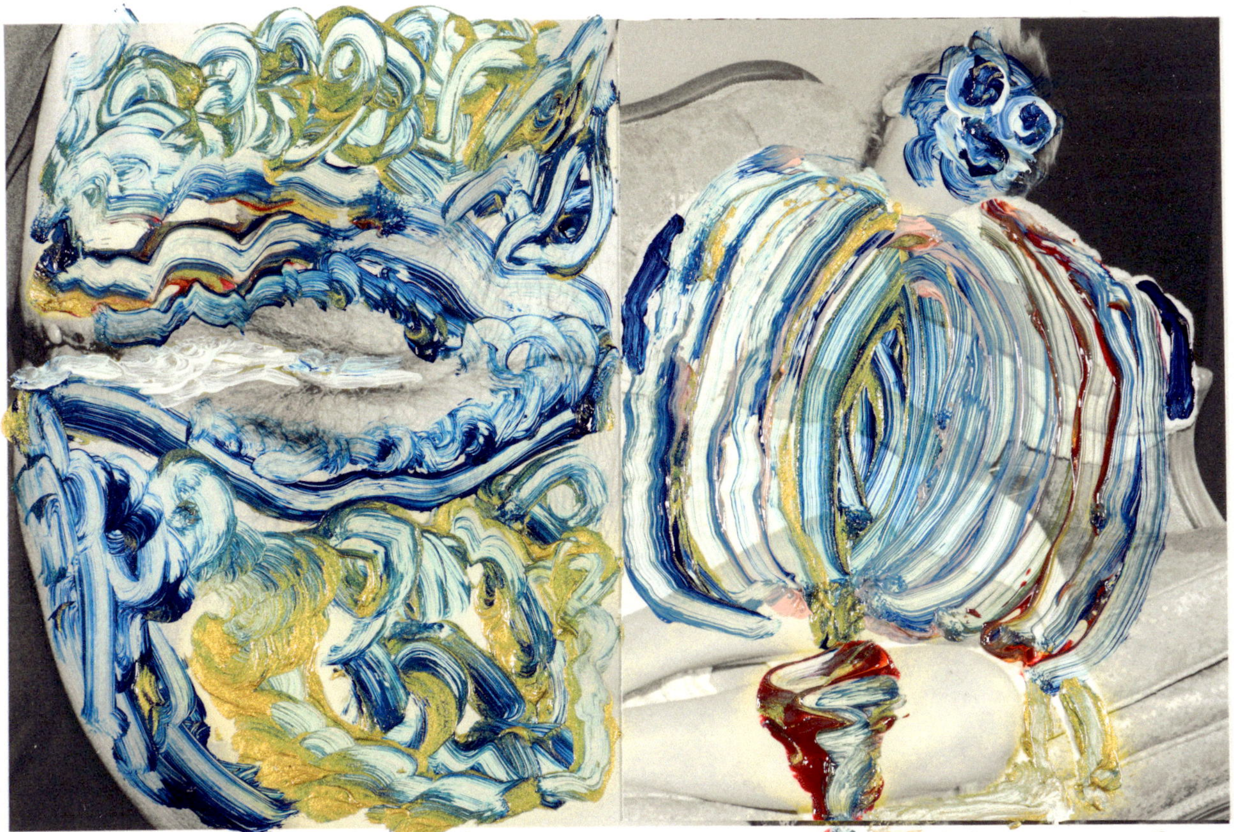

PUDENDAL MOUND & STAPLES   JANUARY 2010

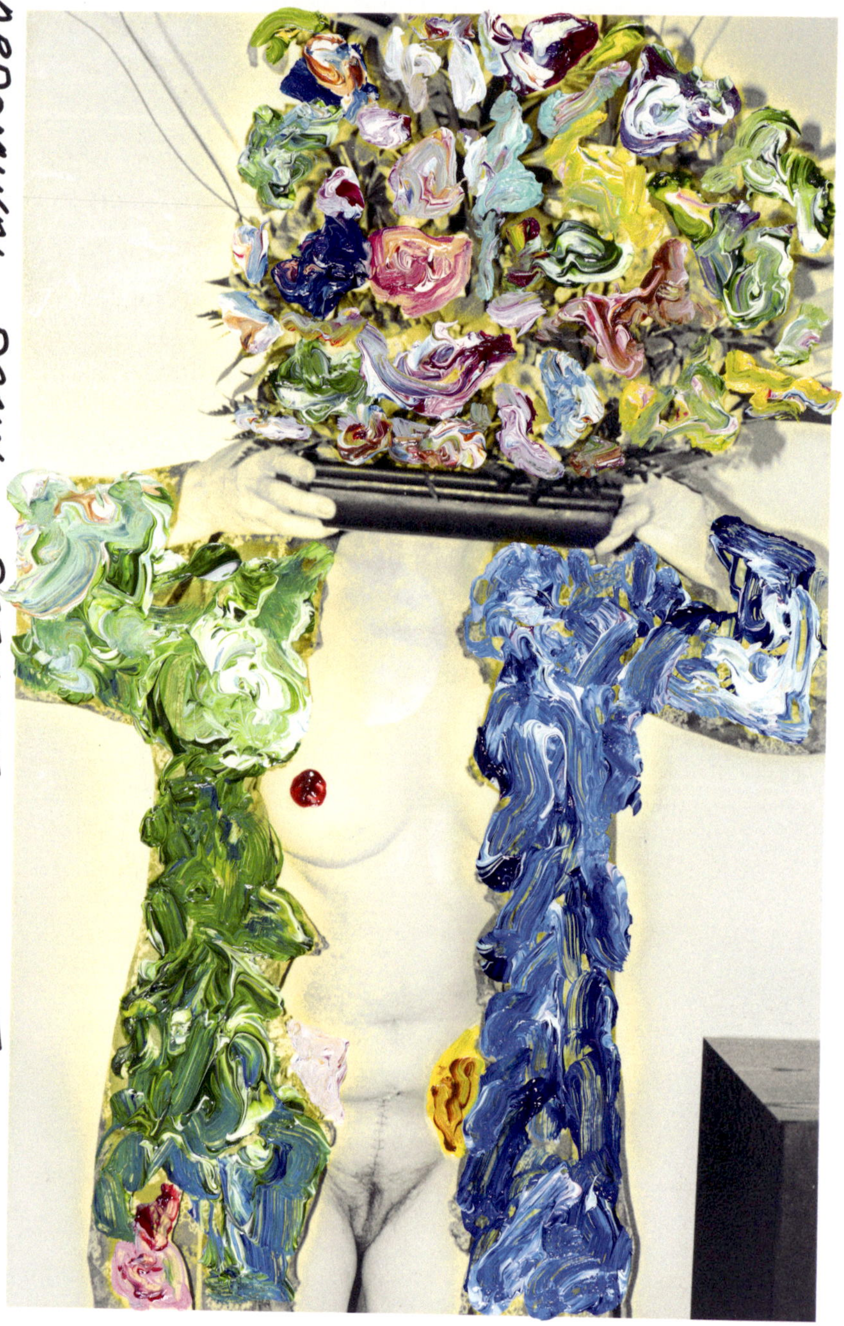

ABDOMINAL DRAIN — DEFIANCE JANUARY 2010

18: Up extra early @ 3:30a to write a lengthy broadcast e-mail to Didy's claque. The disorder weighs heavily. Didy feeling much better, eating soft food, and disconnected from both catheters. Getting used to being with the cat, who now perceives me as an asset.

19: Phone call from Didy @ 7:00a to say that she may be released from the hospital this afternoon. I wheel-chaired her out of the VG and was home by 1:00p. To pharmacy for pain management drugs and to order ostomy supplies. A very sick woman is in this house.

20: Up @ 4a to write e-mail to IJ's friends. Didy weak and fatigued. In quite good spirits though. She enjoyed the snowy day with the fireplace burning and the chicken dinner. first visit from a VON (Victorian Order of Nurses) to dress IJ's back incision (cut from pelvis down to the peritoneum) which has been left open to heal from the inside out. Nurse was a capable woman of the practical straight-ahead Maritime sort. Didy, on high-grade opiates, says the most amazing things at the oddest moments. "You fucked your way through life." "You're the bad, very bad." "You're a little cum machine." "The Meister isn't afraid of a fucking thing." "My beautiful man."

21: Up @ 3:30a, anxious and disoriented. To pharmacy for large order of ostomy supplies. Lovely sunny winter day, white soft snow. Didy sleepy all day. I am beginning to hate, hate, hate living this way.

22: Ingrid Kristina Jenkner (b.1955) 55th birthday. Shopped alone at bakery, coffee roasters, Sobeys, and liquor store. Peggy Mac's turkey casserole for lunch and cod fish chowder for supper. Several photo supply related deliveries. Didy bleeding from her Mesorectal (rear) incision after the nurse changed the dressing. The smell of it is awful. Much laundry.

23: A totally at home day. Didy discharging puss from her rear wound. The nurse showed me how to change the dressing and left a big paper bag of surgical supplies. Washed two loads of bloody bed linen. Very tired. In the midst of it all shot photographs of Didy's incisions, abdominal drain, and ostomy pouch.

24: Woke up angry and driven. Got the morning clean-up going early and made ground up chicken and rice soup. Wrote strongly-worded letter to the Vancouver millionaire and Board Chairman of National Gallery of Canada re. the imminent destruction of Martha's museum (CMCP).

25: To Dr. Russell for a smooth installation of a porcelain crown. Shopped for fish and whiskey. Dr. Jamieson and the visiting nurses consider the bleeding from Didy's rear wound to be part of the normal self-healing process.

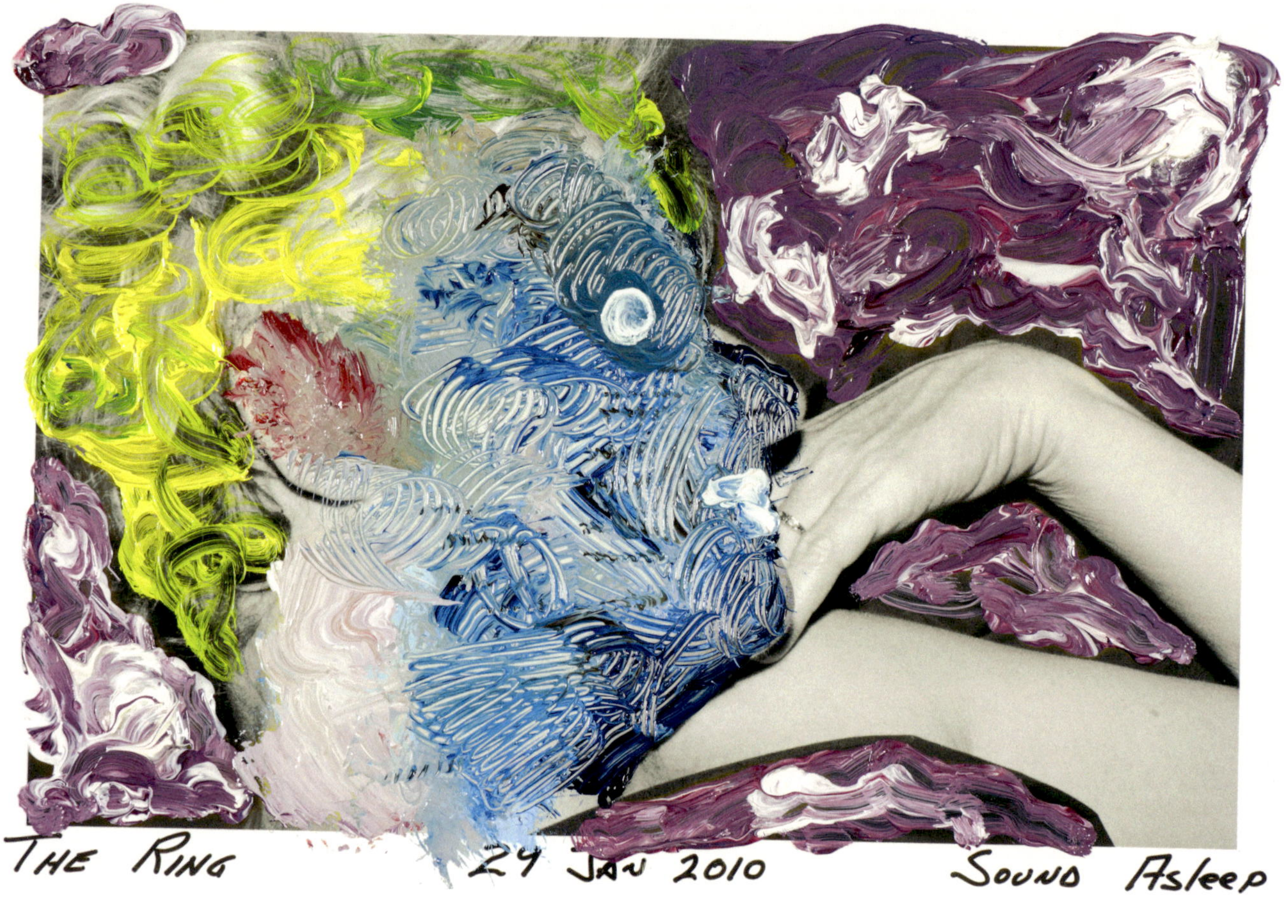

THE RING 24 JAN 2010 SOUND ASLEEP

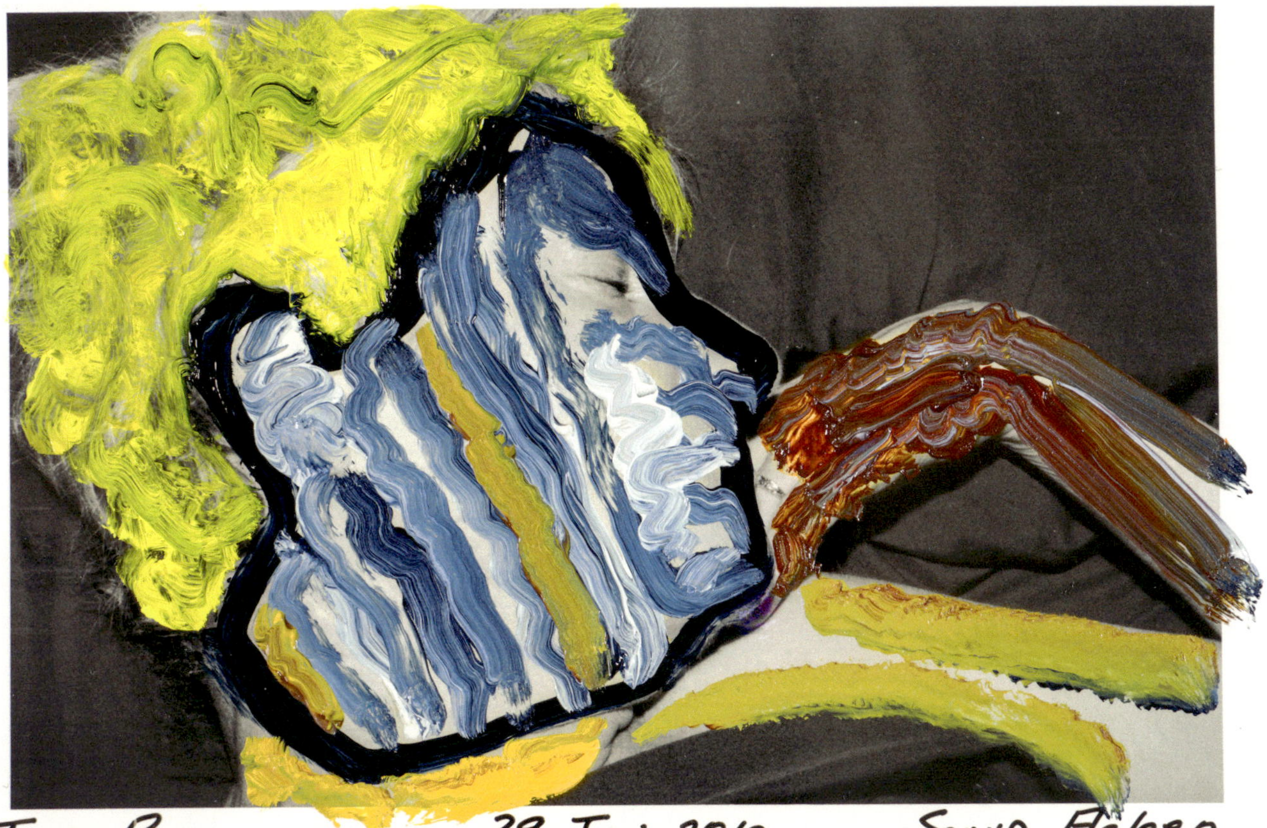

THE RING 29 JAN 2010 SOUND ASLEEP

26: Shopped for groceries and made haddock chowder. Heavy freezing rain and high winds. Didy not at all well—still discharging from perineal wound and in considerable pain. A rough night with IJ with her banging about the house. Finally got the day under way @ 5a.

27: Dr. Jamieson, Victoria General 9th floor @ 2:45p. A sunny and warm +5°c January day. Bundled Didy into a preheated car for the trip to the hospital. Tried to drive as smoothly and slowly as humanly possible so as not to shake Didy. Jamieson made her yelp when he vigorously pulled the drainage tube out of her abdomen. Photographed the procedure.

28: Ordered Sirius satellite radio. Made yet another haddock chowder and then Dijon style chicken breasts for supper. Peter Dykhuis visited in the evening, a kindly and sensitive man. Didy vomited up her supper @ 10a. J.D. Salinger died today.

29: Didy in a lot more pain and looking every inch the part of a sick woman. Fierce winter storm, amazingly the VON got through, robust Maritime women in trucks with able snow tires and always cheerful no matter what. Didy suffering without grace or civility, as is her nature.

30: Cold winter morning. Didy up early to make a bathroom mess for me to clean up. Difficult morning—Didy sullen & in pain. She seemed better when I returned home from shopping perhaps because Peggy Mac dropped off some beef stew and get-well cards from IJ's fawning claque.

31: Didy in a lot of pain & not in a pleasant mood. This always improves with a few large whiskies though. No cooking today—veg stew from Jayne Wark & beef stew from Peggy Mac. Peter Dykhuis visited again, always a relief to see him. As a fellow gallery gatekeeper he instantly draws IJ out of her funk, and he and I have developed a comradely connection.

FEBRUARY 2010

1: Bright white & sunny cold day -18°c. Didy smells so terrible and in a surly and belligerent mood. Will we ever survive this situation intact as a couple? No, maybe we won't. I understand how careless people let things die, bit by small bit. I will fight for us.

2: A calmer night than most after Didy had a fever for a couple of hours. Visit from bubbly Marjorie Simmins bearing fresh flowers and a tonne of cooked food. Didy still struggling with drainage from perineal wound.

ANGER/DESPAIR

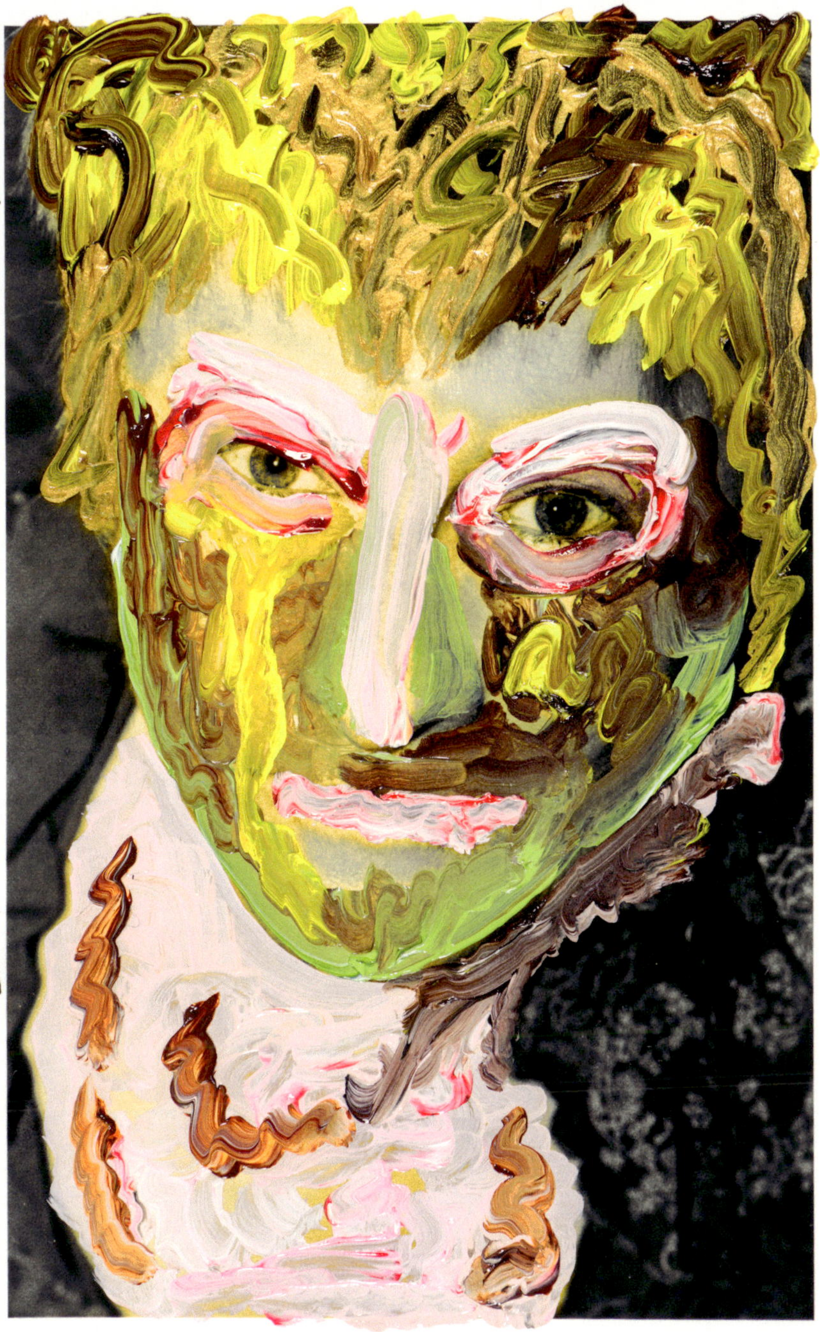

FEBRUARY 2010

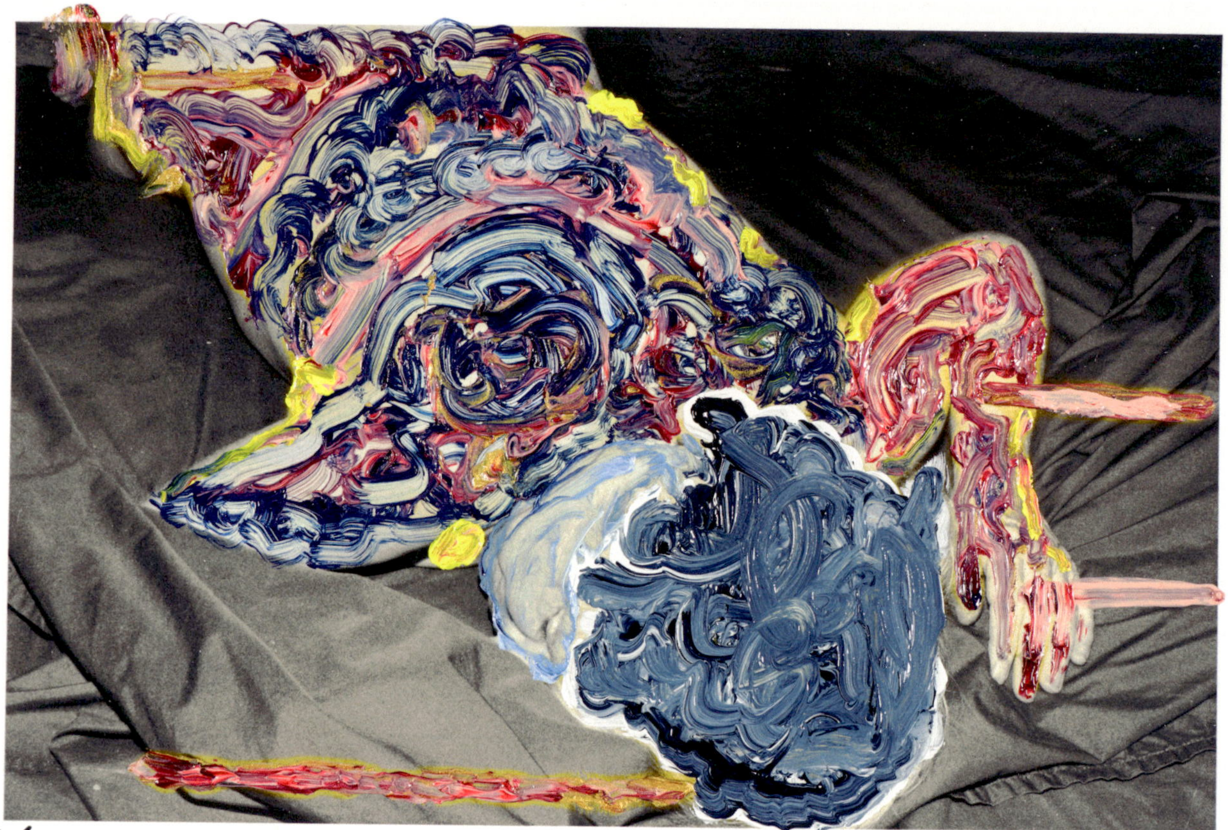

NIGHTMARE 09 FEBRUARY 2010

3: To Victoria General with a beaten down and bedraggled Didy—saw the 'stoma' nurse who made an appointment with Jamieson re. the stench of the ass-end wound. Then home to whiskey, cooking, the VON, and being attacked by the cat.

4: Last night very bad. Didy drunk & nasty. I got up @ 1:30a to find her passed out on the sofa, the stereo blaring, and the poor cat out in the freezing cold. Very angry.

5: 10th anniversary of my father's death, Aubrey Nelson (1913–2000). Tested and activated Sirius satellite radio. Shopped, cooked, cleaned bathroom, and mailed a birthday present to Wolfgang.

6: Opera *Simon Boccanegra* (Verdi). Paper letter to Wolfgang Jenkner (the original retrieved six years later, a year after he died). Didy in extreme discomfort; she advertised the fact constantly, making listening to the opera impossible. Didy cried bitter tears of despair about her now 'ugly' body.

7: Jayne Wark & Peter Dykhuis for a dinner evening. I acknowledge that we socially owe them, but did I really need more domestic work? Felt very nervous & uneasy for no real reason. Didy looked utterly exhausted by evening's end. Cat is sick, pissing in the bathroom sink and bathtub.

8: Didy in pain and not at all gracious. Bulger the cat to the vet for a $400+ fix of her urinary track. I'm sure Bulger is adversely affected by the emotional tension around here. Bulger behaved very well at the animal hospital, charming the Dr. & staff with her endearing ways.

9: Another hard day with Didy in the dirty house. Nothing gets done without a struggle. Ordered flowers from Scrim's in Ottawa for sister Judith's birthday. Hating my life.

10: Cleaned the house. Feel half insane. How did my life sink this low? Will I ever work again. Need to drag myself up, so much more difficult at this age.

11: Wolfgang's birthday. Susanne Swannie thoughtfully brought over a complete chicken dinner for a welcome evening of jollity.

12: A normal day of household tasks and aggravations. There's a building anger that could be turned to creative purposes, I suppose.

13: Opera *La fille du Régiment*. JAR, Judith, called to say she loved the Scrim's flowers. IJ's first outing since the operation, Saturday shopping at Pete's. Pleasant afternoon with the opera and changing of the bed linen. IJ drunk and bad at the end of it.

14: Valentine's Day. A surprise gift from Didy, a crystal heart paperweight. E-mail to Marjorie re. Fiona's, a daughter of the late Richard Simmins, upcoming visit. Peter Dykhuis delivered more cooked food. Didy got really drunk, vomited and acted badly.

15: Appointment with Donna Grant, Licenced Practical Nurse, at Victoria General @ 10:30a. Apparently Didy returned to the bottle after I went to bed last night and was still asleep @ 8a. Mad rush to the hospital. Biopsy report on the surgical debris removed from IJ revealed that the lymph nodes were free of cancer. Extremely good news as the lymphatic system is a major conduit for metastasis. Genital herpes in the rectum was detected.

16: Marjorie and her half-sister Fiona visited @ 2p. How very strange to see little Fiona after ten years. I found it hard to be conversational because I was lost in recollections about her as a little girl and her father, now dead these ten years. Resisted the temptation to bring up the subject of Richard. Marjorie, never lost for words, carried the conversation with hilarious tales of her 50th birthday with her brother (and my faithful correspondent) Geoffrey.

17: Ash Wednesday. Massive winter snowstorm, shovelled four times & cooked wholesome meals. Tension in the house somewhat reduced, perhaps by my own physical fatigue. Solid letter to Peter Schwenger.

18: Solo shopping: bakery, post office, liquor store, gas station, Sobeys. Shovelled more snow. We listened to a new set of CDs, *The Damnation of Faust*. Cooked Didy another solid meal—lots of whiskey.

19: Long confessional letter to Geoffrey. E-mails from a dispirited Miss Heller that I don't honestly know how to reply to. OUP book delayed until April. Unhappy with IJ and the fucking cat.

20: Opera *Ariadne auf Naxos*. Shopped with Didy at Pete's and Crystal & Luckett's wine store. IJ very tired after lunch and slept for hours on my Mum's sofa. Photographed her while asleep. Not a bad day—made beef pasta with roasted red peppers. Didy drunk.

21: Letter to Helen Murphy (Ellen's former girlfriend) re. conditions here. Didy hurt her foot badly while drunk last night. Lovely smooth winter light today, took IJ out for a few shots with the fisheye lens in her new Italian coat. Jayne Wark & Peter Dykhuis for a boozy visit and delivery of Jayne's cooked food—all very upbeat and celebratory.

22: E-mail from Ellen Pierce announcing that Valerie Dean, dear friend and model, has Stage 4 colon cancer, and of course Ellen's own string of current self-inflicted disasters. *CVphoto* seeks back issues for digitization. Photographed Didy's scarred up and stapled lower abdomen.

23: Letter to Angela in England and to Valerie. A much improved day, alone here for the first time in months, IJ to the hairdresser's. Didy returned not feeling well, nasty and aggressive.

24: Unhappy living with Didy and the fucking cat. Another totally wasted day of waiting for nothing. Silence from NSR & Miss Heller—must e-mail them during the night. Spending too much money.

25: Old RBS (Richard Simmins) always said, "Nobody likes an angry man." I must keep this more in the forefront of my thinking. Valerie Dean phoned—she does have Stage 4 rectal cancer (same diagnosis as IJ), but unlike Didy's, it has spread to her liver. How fucking strange is, that Val, whose purity of diet, decades of physical training, and small indulgences, should be the one with a terminal prognosis?

26: Phoned Valerie, who only vaguely sounded like herself. She's in a very bad way with only a short time. Terrible wind and rain storm pounding the house for hours. Heard tremendous banging several times on the roof from cyclonic wind bombs.

27: DAMAGE TO ROOF SERIOUS. Cat still has bladder infection. Didy is to start heavy chemo designed to mop up any residual cancer cells on Monday. No peace on any level. No work & not much thought. What Next?

28: Another ferocious wind and rain storm with the roof already seriously damaged. Roof leaking, water intrusion in the attic. Peter Dykhuis over with more Jayne food to watch Canada win Olympic Hockey gold.

MARCH 2010

1: Didy's 1st post-surgical intravenous chemotherapy @ 1p. Repair crew for emergency temporary restoration of damage to roof. Insurance adjustor inspected the roof and attic. Cat to animal hospital for overnight observation. Another exhausting day. Slept badly.

2: 67th birthday and the worst on record. 2nd powerful chemo @ 1p. Letter opener from Didy. Greetings and mail from Susan and flowers from Miss Heller. Cleaned up backyard storm debris. A grim birthday. Didy started a huge fight in the afternoon. No supper, went to bed @ 6p.

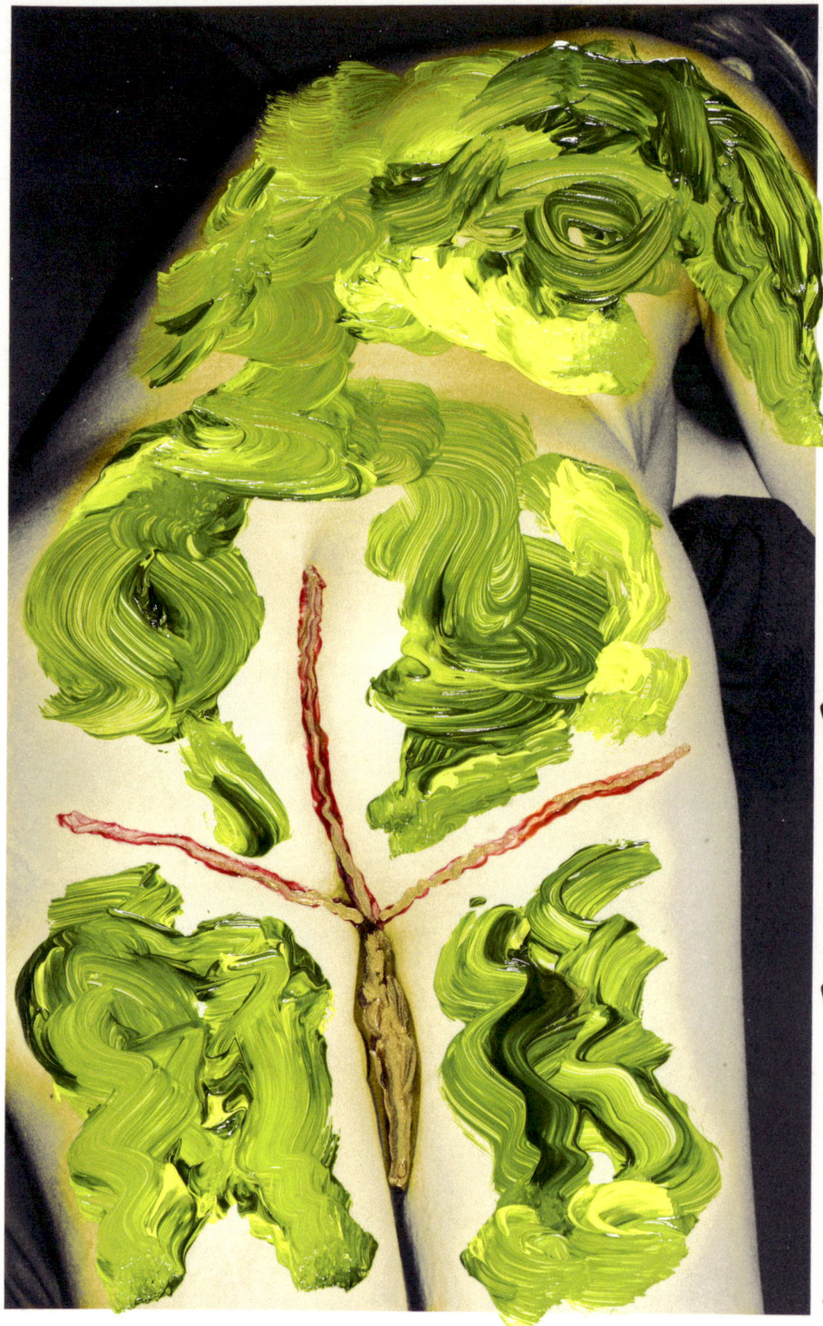

ABDOMINO PERINEAL RESECTION MARCH 2010

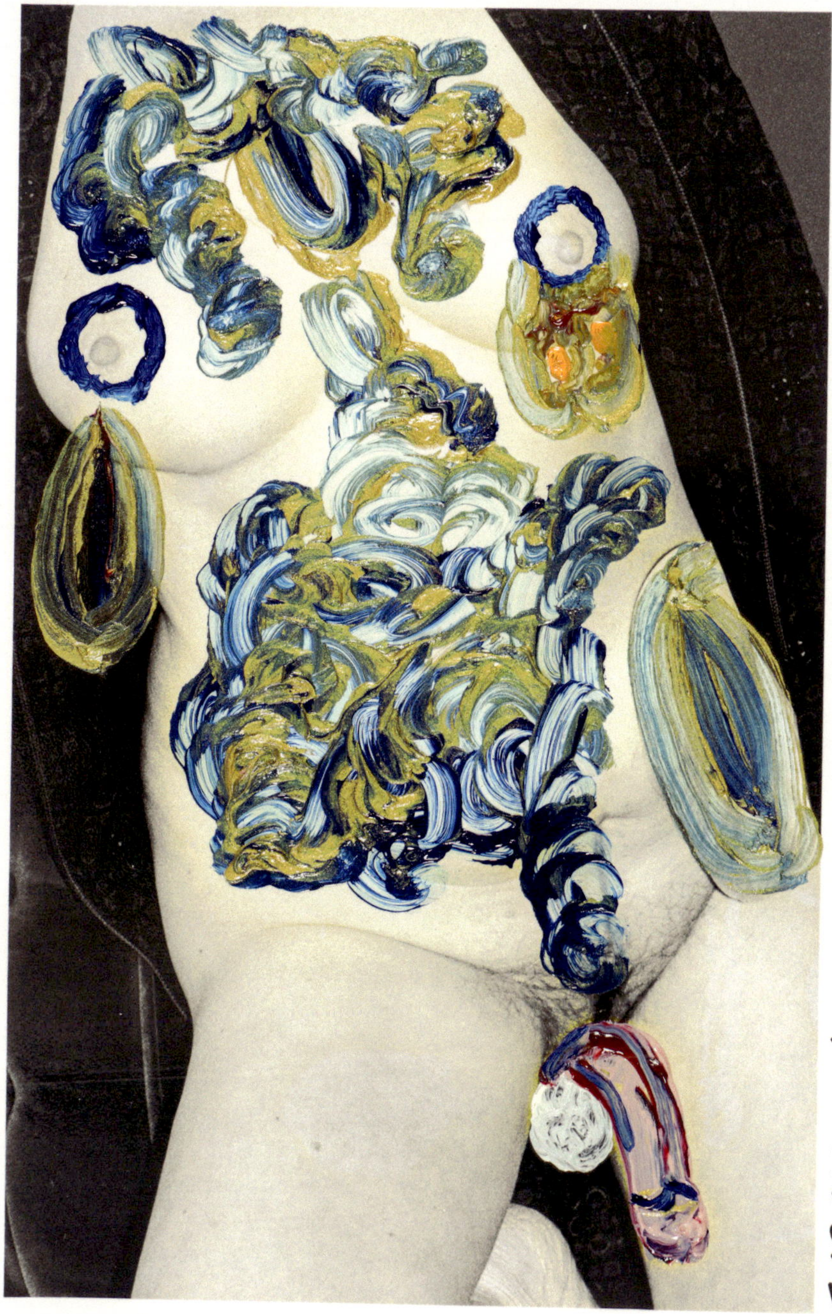

SURGICALLY ALTERED EASTER 2010

3: 3rd massive chemo @ 1p. No one mentioned yesterday's blowout fight. Terribly tired & without hope. Sent thank-you e-mails to Susan, Miss Heller, and Ellen for birthday greetings. House is very dirty again.

4: 4th chemo session @ 1p. A neutral day of drudgery cooking and house cleaning. No reason to believe an improvement is even possible. Wrote a letter to Geoffrey during the night.

5: 5th heavy-duty chemo. Letter from Germany from Robert Wechsler, Angela's decades ago lover. And on this same day a call from Sue Lagasi at the CMCP. What to do with Angela's 1980s letters that I used as the basis for the texts of the *Evidence* series? Dinner out with university dean, Donna Penne, which was very good for us both.

6: My mother, Helen, died on this day five years ago. Woke up in mourning, in grief still. Worked hard in the backyard and took Didy shopping. Tried to be extra good to her. She's immensely fatigued and her food tastes bad to her.

7: Didy not at all well, but well enough to give me a difficult day. Worked on house cleaning, on and off, with no peace or satisfaction. Tension in the house is high. Found time to write Martha & Donigan and Chester Pelkey. Jayne Wark stopped by for wine (Vouvray) and conversation.

8: Didy woke me up in panic, in crisis. Diarrhea poured out of her stoma filling six colostomy bags and sprayed shit all over the bathroom. Then a very rough day with Didy. Worked on the document requested by Jayne Wark.

9: Insurance claim for roof will cover only the patch and attic restoration job. Cleaned myself and the bathroom. Letter to Geoffrey and one received from Helen Murphy. Didy is going to break me.

10: Another brutal day. Didy suffering terribly from chemo side effects. The massive diarrhea is so debilitating. This causes her to be so adversarial especially when drunk. Went to bed without supper again just to avoid her.

11: VW wagon had a tire slashed while parked on the street, likely done by the Italian crime family two doors up the Crescent. So much trouble. Agreed to buy Didy a new washer and dryer. The insurance company's shyster roofing contractor delivered a price quotation of $5480. Geoffrey Simmins in great distress over his delinquent kids.

12: Marjorie Simmins for tea. She's always so cheerful in the best of ways and so generous with her gifts of cooked food. Didy in a better mental space. Ordered a new roof from my preferred contractor at a much lower price.

13: Angela's 55th birthday. Shopped at Pete's downtown. Prof. Randi in free fall. Not a bad day. Worked on preparing for installation of new washer and dryer.

14: Feeling so beset. Needed Valium to get to sleep, then bad nightmares.

15: Woke unrested but calmer. Slow day. Letter from CMCP re. the return of Angela's pink file of the *Evidence* letters (1984–85) for the photo-bunker files.

16: Declared total war on the insurance adjuster by refusing his offer of settlement. Received bullshit letter from the NGC board chair, the luxury homebuilder Michael Audain, re. the annihilation of the CMCP. Time to give up on that. Hardly sleeping at all these days.

17: Men came to replace fibreglass insulation in the attic. Didy's first social outing on her own, lunch with Dr. Randi. Very depressed at being used so badly. Cleaned the house.

18: Bad night, stomach cramps. Felt better in the morning, a cloudy day. Didy uncaring and inconsiderate. Working hard to find a way to live in my own house.

19: Up @ 4a writing to Geoffrey and thinking into the darkness. Unusually smooth day. Insurance adjuster has capitulated with a new settlement. Shopped for supplies to take to Suzanne Swannie's upcoming dinner party. Cooked an excellent supper.

20: A bad start to the day. Didy departed, "to get the car washed," but really to smoke cigs. Made large German potato salad for the party and shopped for Atlantic salmon & oysters.

21: Cooked with Suzanne Swannie in her kitchen a dinner party for seven. We worked together as if we'd done it for years: broiled salmon, oysters on the half-shell, and potato salad. Everyone enjoyed themselves. Up @ 4a to write Valerie, who I fear is a goner.

22: My BIO workmate, Garon Awalt, over @ 10a to help install a 240 VAC receptacle for the new clothes dryer. Quite hungover and depressed. Didy annoying and thoughtless. Cleaned downstairs after manhandling dismantled old washer & dryer out to the street.

23: Sears delivered washer & dryer in a heavy & cold rain. Much dirt to clean up. Didy secretly smoking again. Long and moving letter from Geoffrey Simmins.

124: Cleaned the downstairs after a muddy installation of the washer and dryer. Tested both, seemed OK. Cooked and cleaned as usual. Scavengers took away old units.

25: Life could be so much better than this and should be given all the work that went into building it. No reason at all to think that this awful way of living will go on indefinitely.

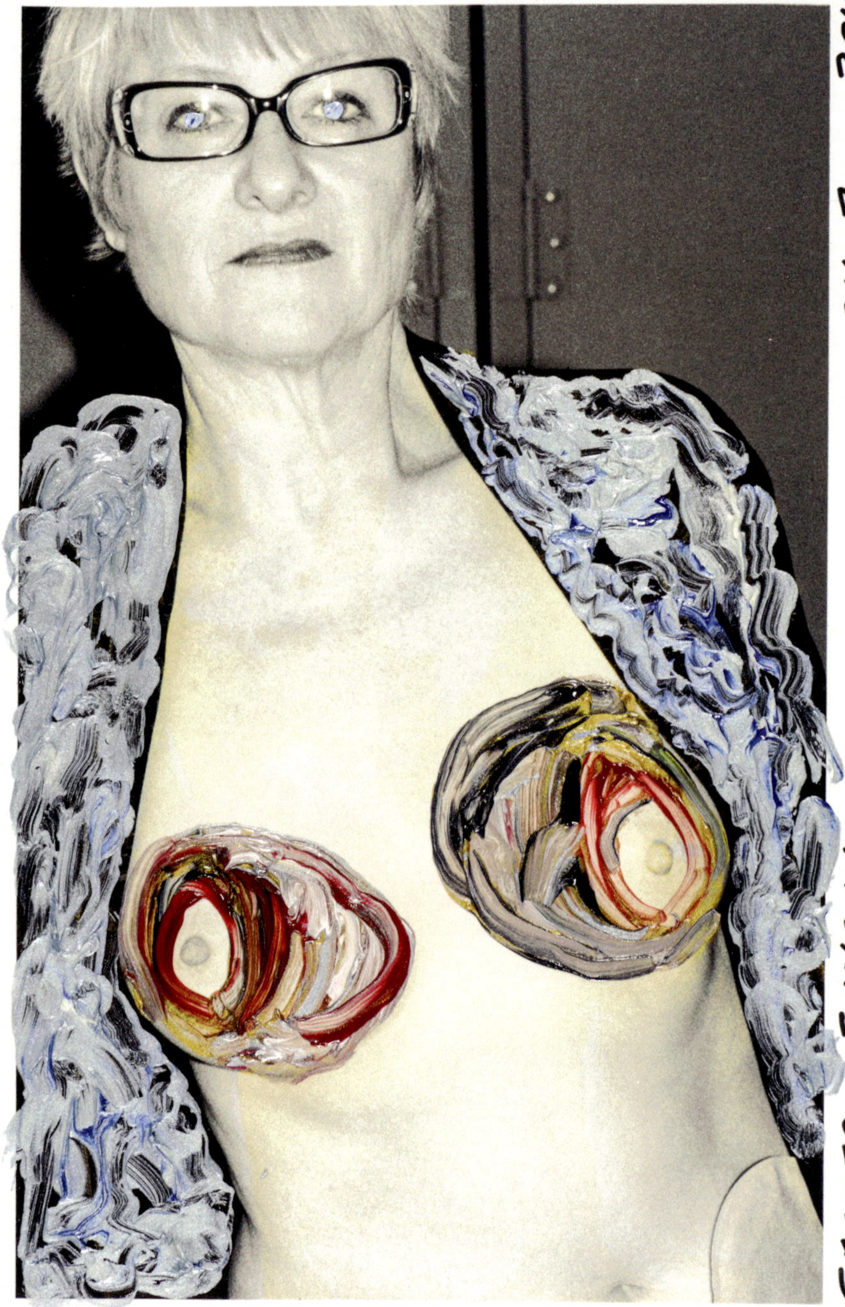

EASTER SUNDAY 04 APRIL 2010

26: Stormy March day with thoughts only of photo work not done and for company not available. FedEx delivered the Angela file from the CMCP. Spooky to see the old letters with all that painful personal history.

27: Tired after a bad night of dreams. Caught up on correspondence. Strange no word from Angela yet this year. Made roasted chicken soup and pork tenderloin for supper.

28: Palm Sunday. Wrote letter to NSR & to Donigan. Long, of course, e-mail from Chester in Saskatoon. Quite a happy day. Shopped with Didy at Pete's in Bedford. Ran into an old colleague from BIO, Nelson Rice, in the parking lot. Cooked prime rib roast with white asparagus in cream sauce.

29: Woke up wanting to fuck and be sucked. Morning exercises with Didy, then to hospital for a long nerve-wracking session of waiting. Didy's white blood cell count insufficient to resume chemotherapy this week.

30: Up @ 4a writing and thinking. Didy posed for nudes. Then accepted an invitation for coffee without telling me where she was going.

31: Didy in a bright mood buoyed by a visit from two dykes from New Brunswick. Insurance company has caved and will pay the full cost for a replacement roof. Gave Didy her first bill for her half of common household expenses. She is feeling better.

APRIL 2010

1: "Val's Story," an 8-page e-mail supposedly narrating her journey in cancer-land, but in reality a lot of self-deluding New Age babble. Drinking gallons of beet and carrot juice will not stop stage-IV colon cancer. Val's strange husband, Don, sent me a copy of his letter explaining their situation to his parents, which made slightly more sense.

2: Thinking of LFH at 8 Graham St, NSR at Thelma Ave (Toronto), and Val & Don all lost to my reality. Made Shepherd's pie while Didy schmoozed with 'artists'.

3: Opera *Aida*. Jayne Wark for dinner. Sleeping with Didy for an hour or so each morning. Had our first joint shower this morning. Pleasant shopping together at Pete's. Made scalloped potatoes and baked ham.

4: Easter Sunday. Inching closer to getting my cock into Didy's cunt. Lovely warm day, worked in the yard with Didy. A general improvement in mood and outlook.

5: Warmth of the sun on a spring-like day. Didy in a good mood. Listened to *Tannhäuser* on the satellite radio. Feeling very horny, spring fever.

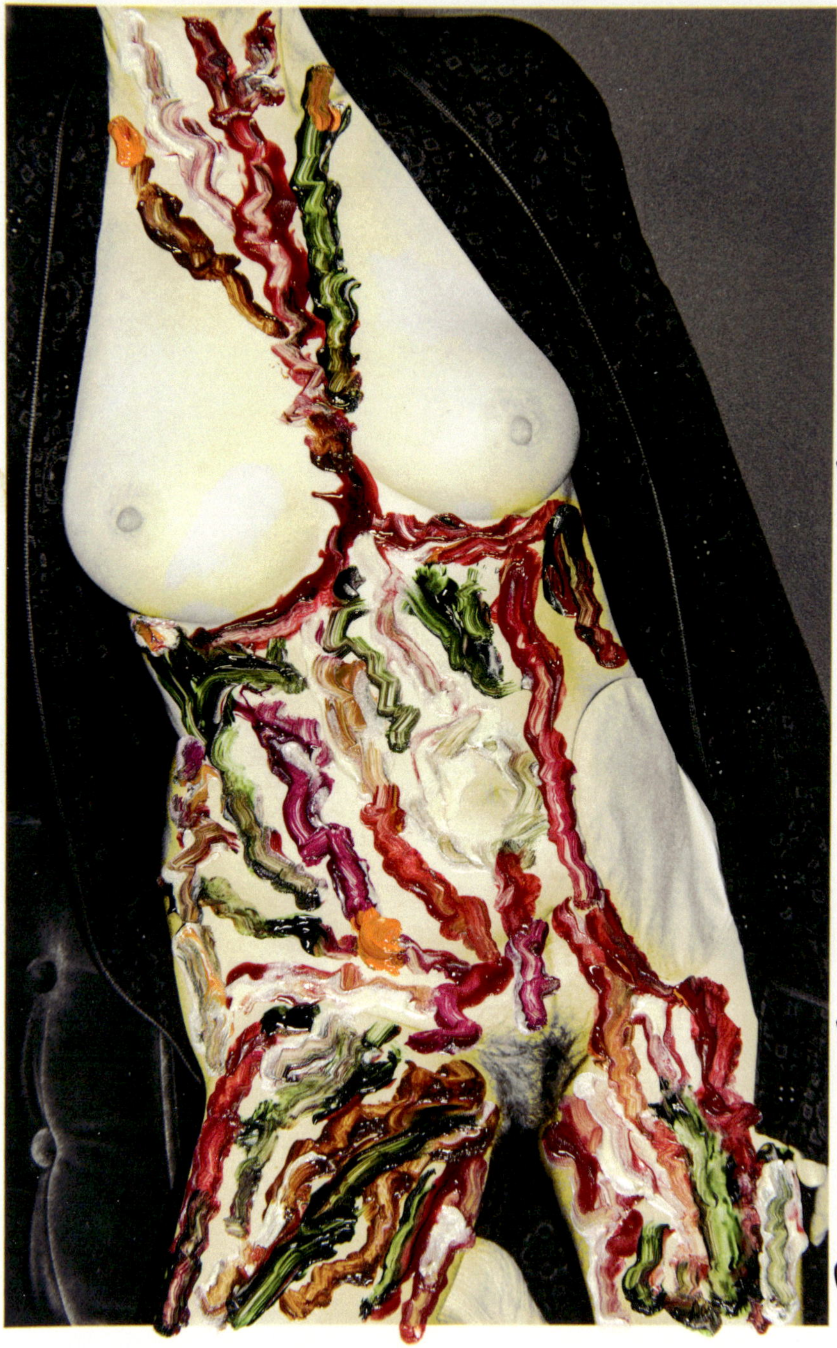

PRINTED SILK EASTER 2010

6: Chemotherapy resumed after blood analysis indicated a higher white blood count. Long day in the chemo ward 10:30a to 4:30p. Arrived home tired and nervous.

7: Quick chemo run to the VG. Cooked a solid and nutritious supper. Didy quite tired, but became amorous when in bed. We attempted sexual intercourse, but penetration not yet possible, she finished me by hand.

8: Smooth chemo run. Ordered a ceramic Dutch oven. Didy's mood very good. Miss Heller e-mailed ranting on in a semi-psychotic state about her life with Tim, 'The Woofer'.

9: Non-penetrative sex in the morning, then exercised together. Completed and mailed IJ's income tax return. Chemo was quick today. Supper of ham and sweet potatoes, then an episode of Rumpole.

10: Opera *Die Zauberflöte*. To VG for the last infusion of this round of heavy chemo, and because it was a Saturday in the Haematology Ward. The nurses were ultra careful and meticulous, each checking everything independently and signing a form to that effect. Shopped at Pete's downtown and cooked while the 'flute' played at the Met. Didy tired but in good spirits.

11: Phoned sister Judith in Victoria, BC. Made pot of ham and pea soup. Party in the Gottingen Street apartment of Sarah Hollenberg, somewhat of a Passover affair.

12: 3 photocards from Geoffrey about his grad school days in Toronto with Jayne Wark and his demon-bitch lover Leslie Korrick. Didy has moved to the dark precipitous side of a post-chemo crash.

13: Cleaned the house. Becoming resentful of domestic drudgery. 2 more photocards from Geoffrey about his cock-teaser lover Leslie's 'all show, no go' sexual manipulations.

14: Shopping for home improvement materials at Kent Lumber. Worked in the yard with Didy, who unknown to me was feeling very bad, the post-chemo blow-back. I was harsh with her about her dirty ways and then I was so sorry. Insurance cheque on the way.

15: Pathetic and heart-rending phone message from a dying Val Dean. How can I help her when I'm so overburdened with IJ? Didy told me that her peritoneal incision has opened due to last week's attempts at sexual intercourse. I owe Revenue Canada $2002 this year.

16: Glynis Humphrey and her Welsh corgi for lunch at Tangmere. A fine boozy afternoon until Glynis stupidly locked us out of the house when she and IJ went out for cigs. The miser-hoarder people across the street have spare keys, but of course they couldn't find them. Then had to drive over to Garon's (one of the few responsible people I know) for his keys.

17: Opera *La Traviata* (ravishing performance). Shopping at Pete's on a pleasant winter-like morning. E-mails of substance from Chester Pelkey, Liane Heller, and Don Reider (on Val's condition). He demanded to see me; I definitely don't want to see him, knowing he'll ask me for money. I don't see much happiness out there these days.

18: Rain and wet snow. Wanting to fuck but Didy not nearly well enough. Raucous drunken evening with Jayne & Peter that pleasantly rolled on until midnight.

19: Third attempt at post-operation fuck. Didy in too much pain to accept full penetration, so I ejaculated in her outer lips. Both of us quite hungover. Snow still hanging around. Purchased barbeque on Didy's orders.

20: Mailed income tax return at regional post office, then across the street to the Brooklyn Warehouse to host Marjorie and Silver Donald Cameron for an uproarious lunch. Received insurance cheque for $6860.79. Didy in good humour, as am I.

21: A bad day in my head. Angry with Didy, her selfishness and sense of entitlement. No joy in anything. Why be here at all? Feel like the little backyard squirrel, I too hang onto twigs.

22: Wonderful warm +17°C spring day. Mood on the opposite swing from yesterday. Happy card from Marjorie. Placed order for books and DVDs. Cooked Teriyaki steaks and braised Brussels sprouts.

23: St. George's Day. Sea fog envelopes the neighbourhood. Letter from NSR. A quiet insular day undercut by sexual frustration. Cooked two full meals and cleaned up. Didy seemed happy with "a nice life."

24: Bulger the cat is sick again. The poor thing must be also suffering from the atmosphere around here. She had extreme diarrhea and needed extensive cleaning out on the deck. Tempers flared. Then to shop and calm down. Cooked pot roast in new French clay baker.

25: Didy rampaging through the house, issuing directives, and oppressing me. Thinking seriously of killing myself to escape this terrible trap.

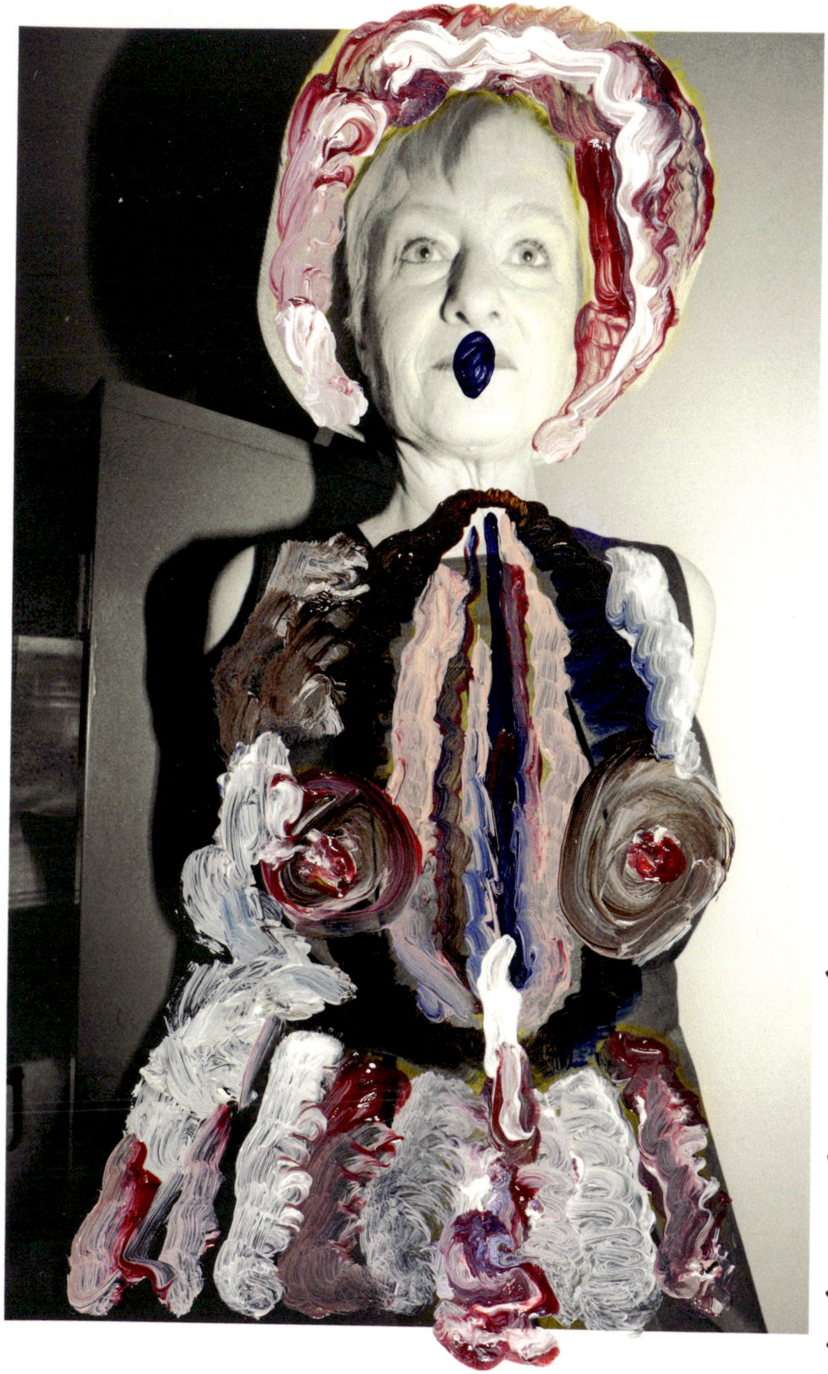

Spring 2010

Who Am I Now?

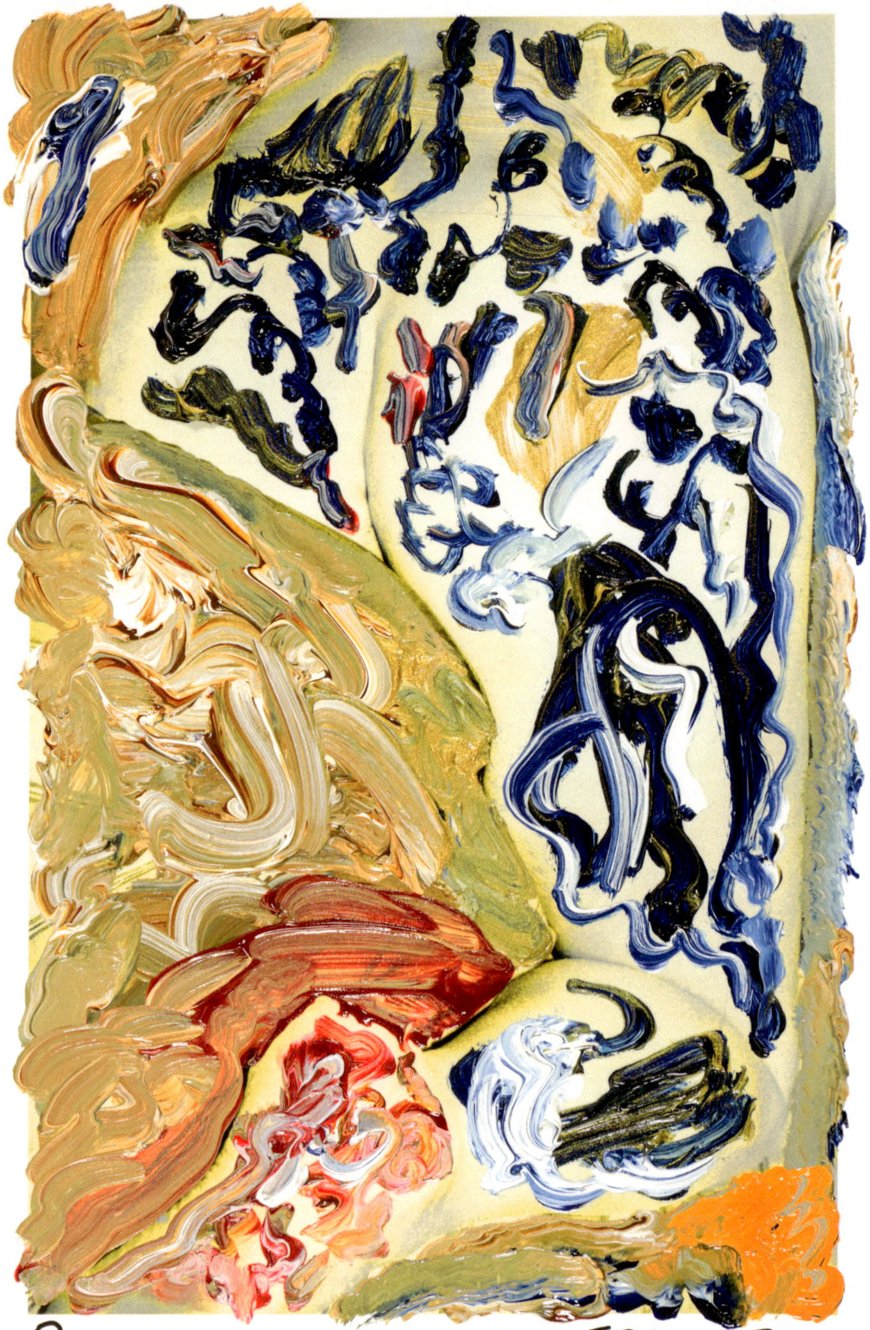

PROCTECTOMY SPRING 2010

26: At last fucked Didy with full penetration of her now even tighter low-riding cunt. Didy visited Randi, the crazy Mount professor.

27: My old VW Golf, Didy's adopted car, at the dealer's for routine service. Quiet day with Didy. Roasted chicken in a French style. To bed early.

28: Morning stand-up hand-job. Randi Warne using Didy to no good purpose. I will protect Didy from this injurious influence. Cars are both spring tuned up.

29: Shopping trip for barbeque tools and coffee. Trying to enjoy this good week of Didy's time at home. Dr. Randi has been cut off, phone messages unanswered.

30: 65th anniversary of the suicides at the Voßstraße bunker. To Pete's for first fiddlehead greens of the spring. Didy initiated penetrative sex this morning, full lusty and balls-deep. A day of spectacular atmospheric effects. No mail & no phone calls—Randi the lunatic silent.

MAY 2010

1: To Annapolis Royal on a beautiful spring day. IJ visited the Lucky Rabbit pottery in her capacity as gallery director, where she bought me an elegant coffee mug. Also we dropped in on Katie Belcher's drawing show. Dinner and overnight in Digby. Didy forgot her purse at the restaurant.

2: Retrieved Didy's purse at the restaurant @ 10:30a, then drove home in a storm of spring insects. Cooked a very good pork roast in new French pot.

3: To Victoria General for third round of heavy chemotherapy infusions. IJ's white blood cell count too low for chemo. Must wait another week to proceed. Didy looking very old and tired at times and I'm sure I do as well. Plain supper and DVD watching.

4: Bright fresh day. Assembled new barbeque. Grand letter from Geoffrey re. his trip to Chicago where he met his old girlfriend, the man-killer Leslie. Didy OK.

5: Woke up with the urge to fuck, but Didy was messed-up with the colostomy apparatus. Didy now openly smoking. That made me visibly depressed. Used barbeque for first time, but was too depressed to eat the food.

6: Woke in better spirits. Didy gave me a long slow hand job. Roof shingles arrived on a pallet for next Monday's roofing job. Didy to the university for a meeting to schedule her return to work.

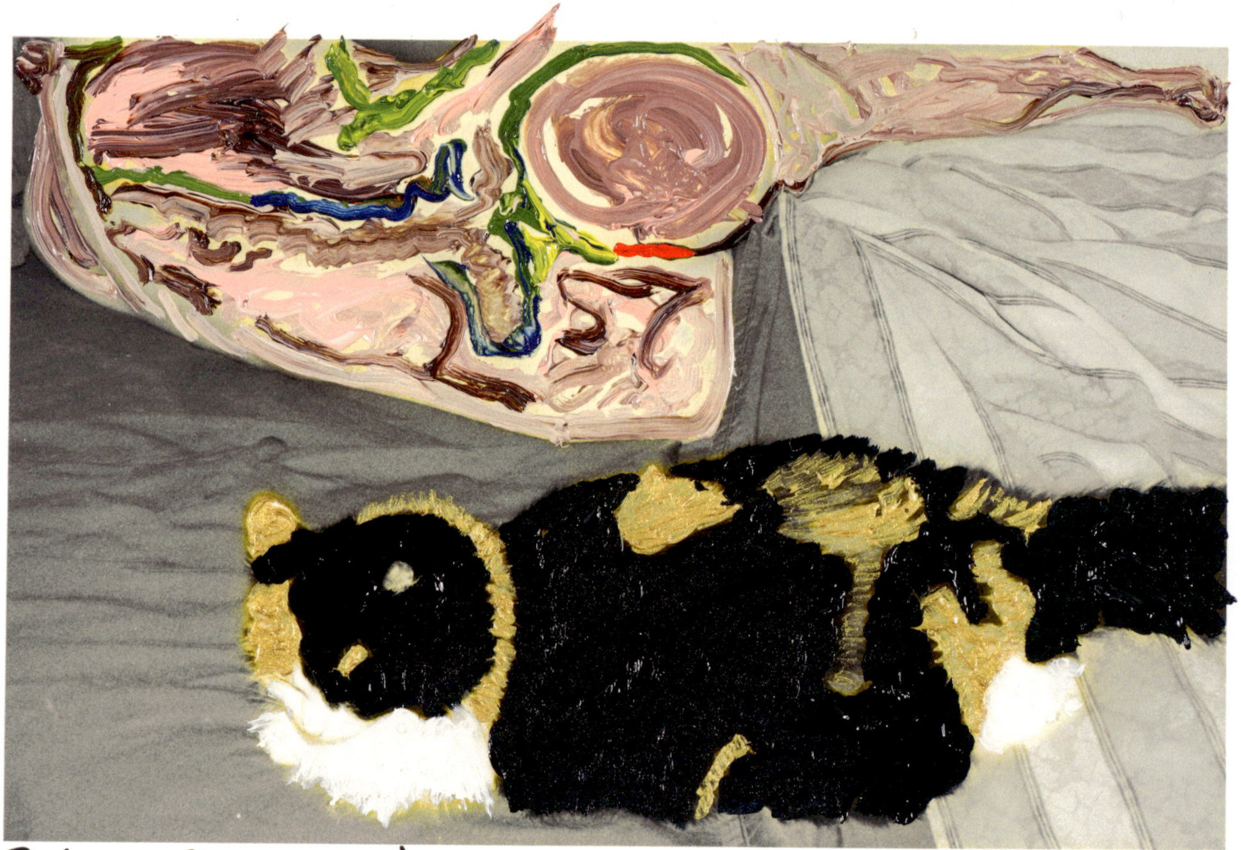

BULGER (1999-2016) SPRING 2010

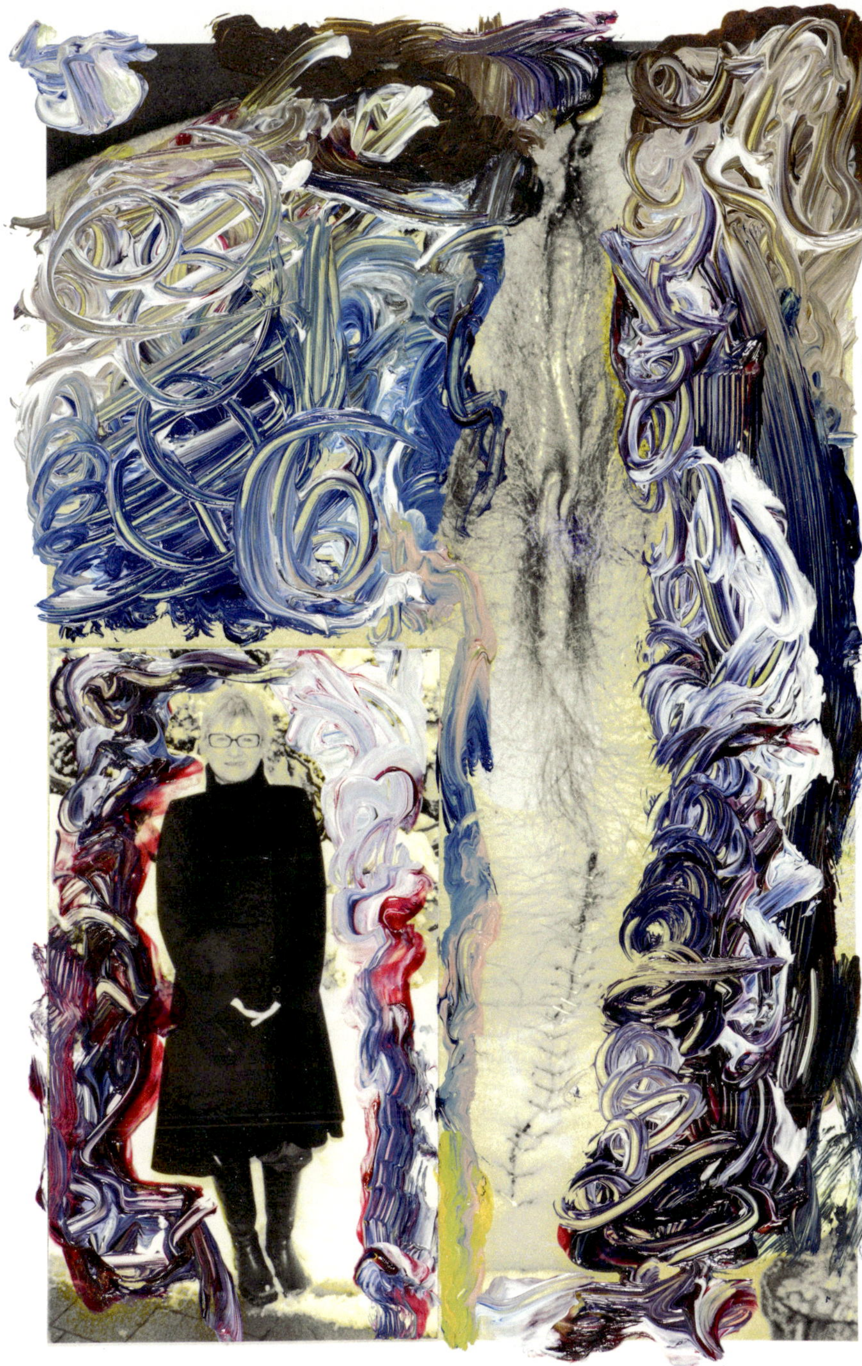

PINK FOLDS & SURGICAL TRENCH 2010

7: Greek financial crisis caused deep stock market plunge. Barbequed chicken breasts. A slow day but not unpleasant. Feel an urgent need to resume photo work after almost a year's hiatus.

8: Bathroom tiles came away from a portion of the wall. Wrote a letter to Angela in England. Barbequed steaks. Tenderly fucked Didy in the middle of the night.

9: Long phone conversation with Martha and Donigan. Drank all day and evening. Elegant dinner party at Peter & Jayne's.

10: Chemo @ 10a. White blood cell count satisfactory. Insurance cheque not accepted by the bank. New roof completely installed in six hours by a double work crew.

11: Chemo run to the VG @ 9:30a. Mailed insurance cheque back with a stern letter. Shopped for food at Pete's and wine at C&L, then home to cook and wash. Didy to gallery for her first 4-hour workday.

12: Chemo @ 10a. Very tired. Started a birthday letter to NSR. In a depressed mood when Didy came home out of sorts and unfriendly. Started the night downstairs but returned to Didy's bed for a clumsy abortive sexual encounter.

13: Will today be better than yesterday? Quick chemo trip to the VG @ 10:30a. Cleaned things around the house. Didy dead tired by chemo and 4 hours at the gallery. There's no need for her to work when still in cancer treatment.

14: Last heavy chemo infusion @ 8:30a of this the third post-operation round. Didy obnoxious then departed for the Mount. She made gratuitous requests for changes to the house while herself never lifting a finger for anything around here.

15: Didy has decided to see how far she can push me around today, in all the small ways she knows so well. If we had separate living spaces I would simply go home, but I don't have a home anymore and never will. There are only two solutions: suicide and divorce, I sometimes think but don't believe.

16: Not so much in turmoil today. Grilled salmon and drank moderately. Pondered the upcoming changes when Didy goes back to work full time.

17: New camera bag with 'GDS' embroidered in black on black. Lovely day outside, but I'm depressed. Income tax assessment OK. Grilled steaks and felt better when Didy got home.

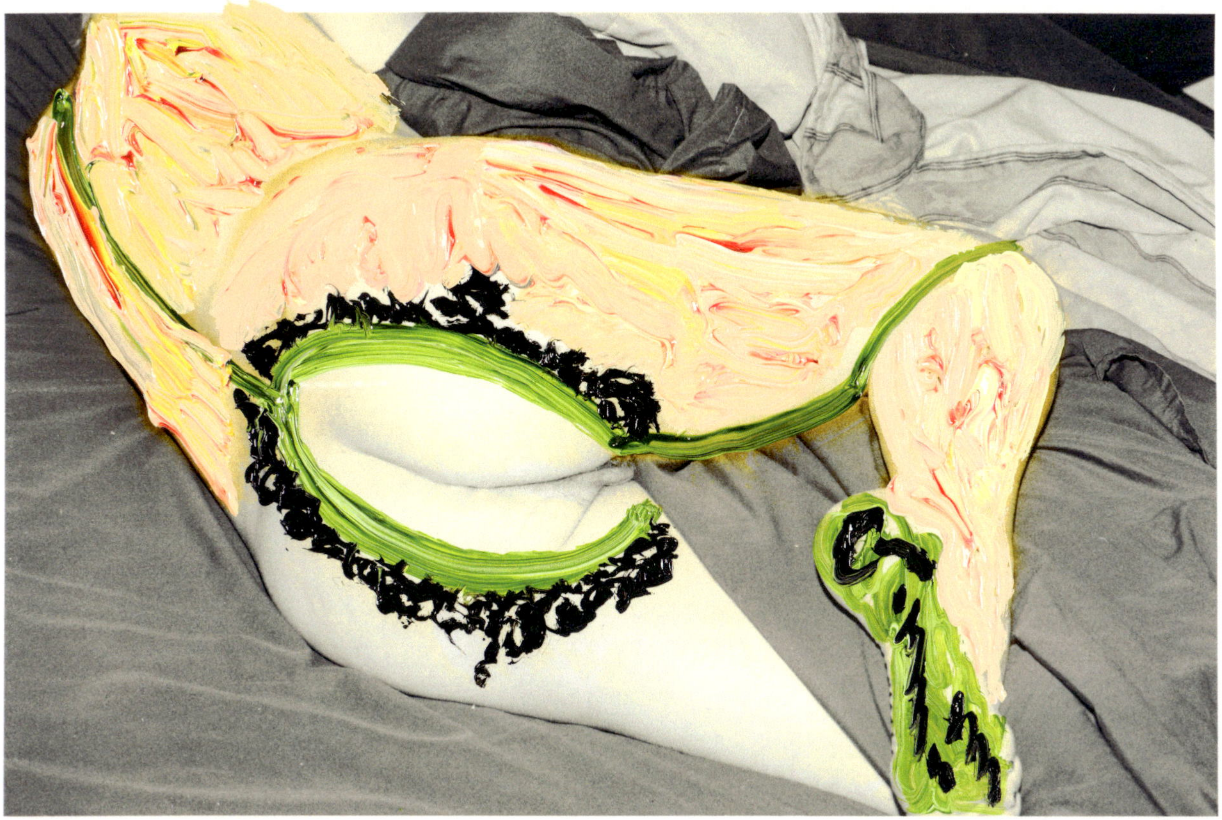

SANS ANUS SPRING 2010

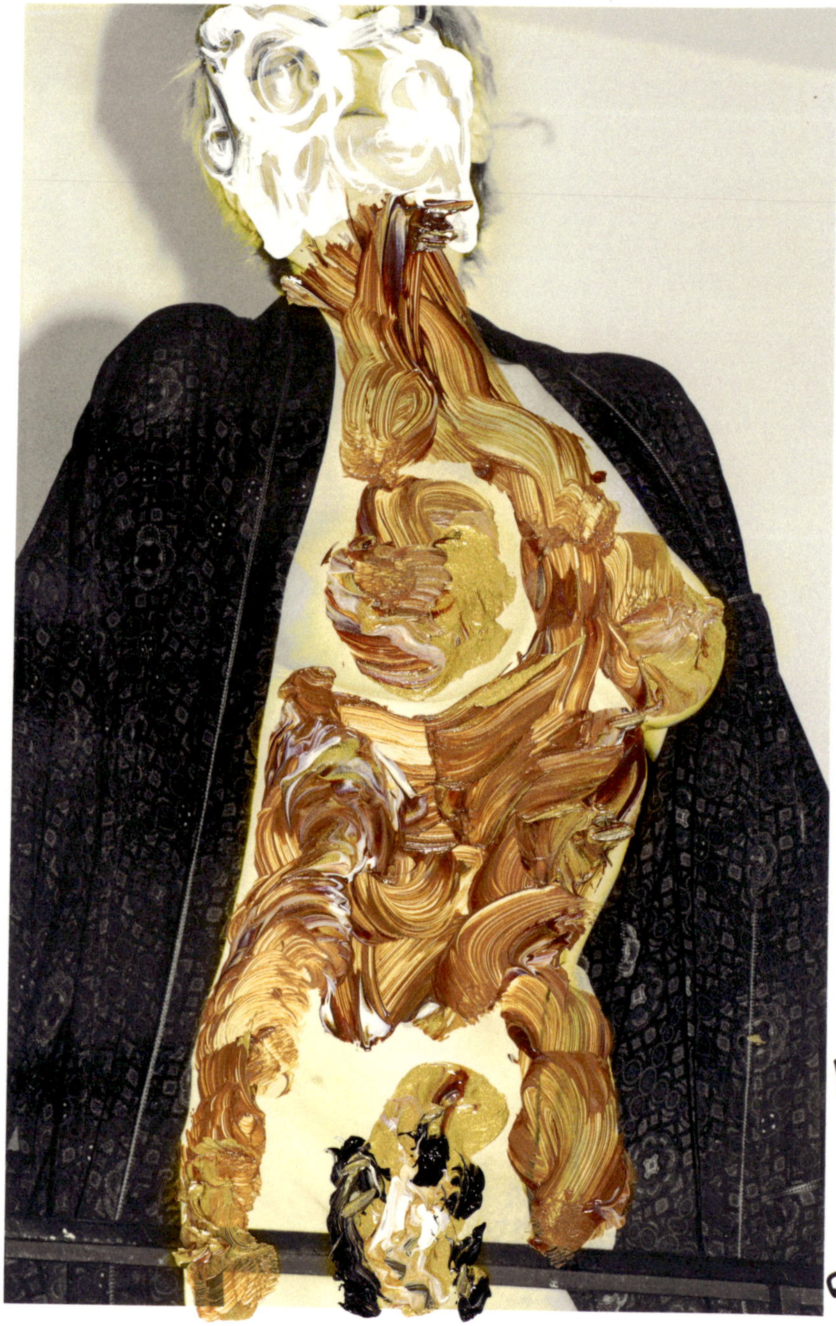

RISING ANXIETY

MAY 2010

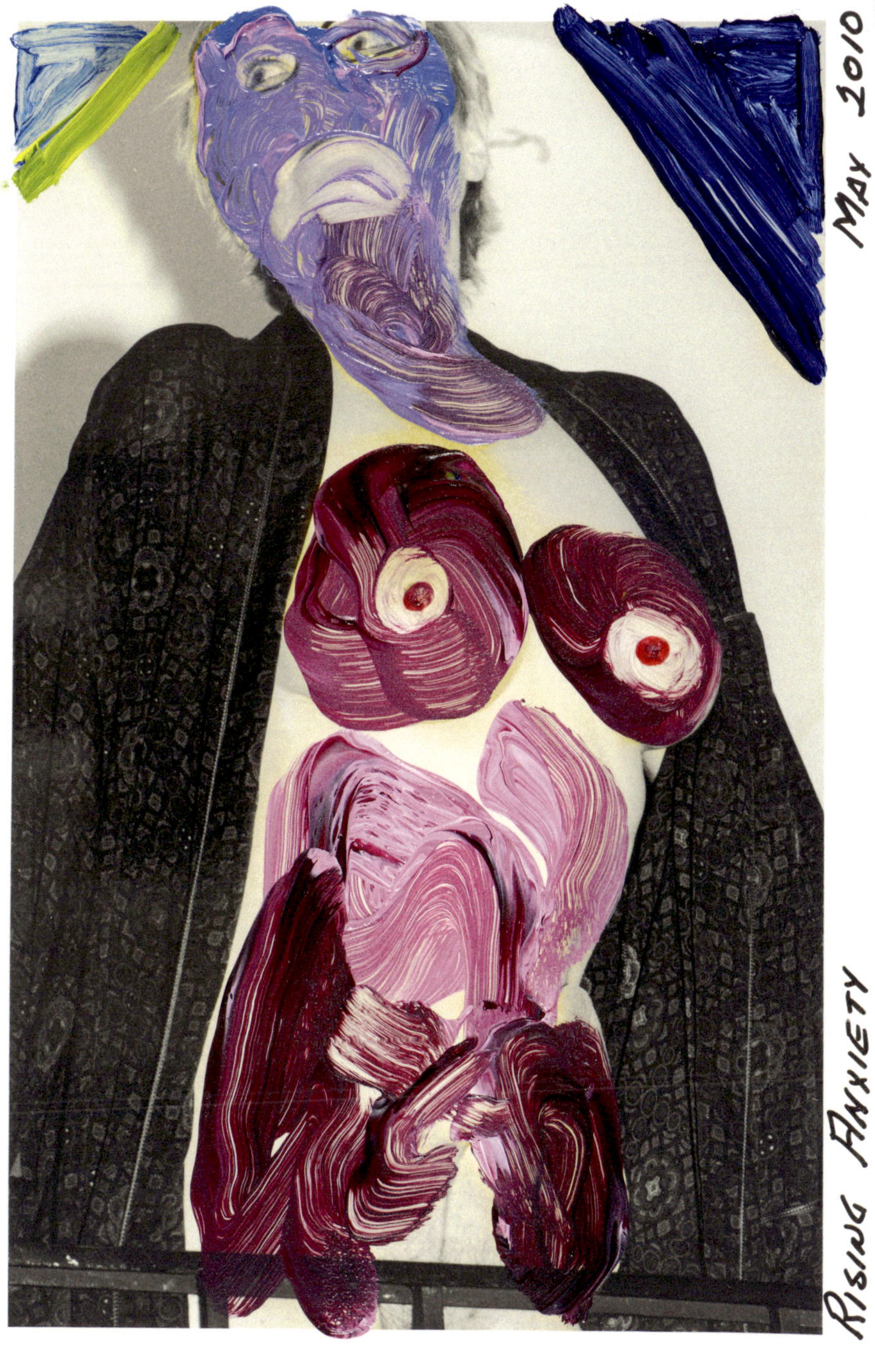
Rising Anxiety
May 2010

18: Contracted to have bathroom tiles fixed. Phoned Light Impressions re. order for photo supplies; they charged my credit card, but have not shipped the goods (and never did). Updated my photo cv. Walked in the sun with Didy.

19: Visited poor Valerie Dean at the VG 11th floor chemo ward. I walked right by her in an infusion chair and had to ask a nurse where she was. I simply did not recognize one of my oldest friends. Her spirit is still vibrant but her body is wasting away. The four weeks she was given have been revised upward to a 30% chance of living 5 years.

20: Loving tender letter from Val and an ominous note from her husband Don. Woke sexually aroused, but Didy wasn't interested in my hard cock. Cooked and cleaned as usual.

21: Resentfully cleaned the house upstairs, feeling exploited and unappreciated.

22: Cleaned the house downstairs, in another angry mood. Loath living together with IJ and the dirty cat. Death and divorce never far from my thoughts.

23: In a better frame of mind today. Willing, for the day, to be the domestic servant. Prepared food for tonight's dinner party with Peter and Jayne. German potato salad, white asparagus with sauce, and grilled Atlantic salmon.

24: Victoria Day. Hungover and stayed in night gown all day. Barbequed twice and cleaned the kitchen three times. Very warm spring day. Didy not that well and uninterested in intercourse even after I masturbated her to a climax.

25: Phoned Light Impressions again re. screwed up photo order; this is going to end badly. Quite impossible to make anything positive happen. Didy combative; I slept downstairs.

26: A more productive day, oh so slowly creeping back into photo work. Worked on the mailing list. Wrote the Reverend Dr. in Calgary. Why is sexual desire so overwhelming these days?

27: Insurance company issued new cheque. I did not attend Miss Heller's book launch at the Company House with Dr. Astrid Brunner present—poetry concerning the evils perpetrated by me when I 'dumped' her for Ingrid.

28: Didy woke up in a randy way. Told me to stay in bed while she prepared herself in the bathroom. Then wrapped her legs around my torso as I thrust all the way inside her. Worked on correspondence and texts for the Xmas photocard mailout. Barbequed ribs and drank too much, all in a rather good mood.

29: Didy woke up sexually aggressive and lavishly exhibitionistic. She has resumed her practice of reaching down under her buttocks to squeeze my scrotum when she's ready to accept the ejaculate. Later an attack of back pain; no wonder there. Cooked prime rib roast served with New Brunswick fiddlehead greens and new potatoes.

30: Didy woke me up by deciding to have an impromptu and private party for herself and the cat in the middle of the night. I joined the party and after a few restorative drinks came up to speed. She dragged me down onto the old India living room carpet and had her way with me, riding upright on my erection.

31: A lost day, but why shouldn't it be? Didy in a mood of thought-free jollity and given to displays of amorous provocation.

JUNE 2010

1: Didy's 1st full day back at the gallery. Very troubled about restarting my photo practice all over again. Cooked, cleaned, and shopped instead.

2: A really hard purple-headed cock deep into Didy's cunt. A better mood today. Still waiting for insurance cheque. A pleasant late afternoon when Didy got home. Barbequed slab of roast beef. A video watching night.

3: Busy domestic day: laundry, post office, cleaned grout from old bathroom tiles, mowed lawn, set up new toaster oven, and made supper. Val Dean and Miss Heller silent.

4: Major fight with Didy last night triggered by her gross rudeness. Eventually patched things up @ 2:30a and then I wanted to fuck which was allowed. Insurance cheque $6860.79.

5: Strong steady full-depth sex. Another major shopping at Pete's, crown roast of pork & expensive wine. Gloomy and depressed, can't shake off bad thoughts about marriage to Didy. But as she often says, we married late in life with little tolerance remaining. She's secretly smoking again. It shakes one's nascent trust.

6: Bad nightmares about graduate school oral math exams, even though I received straight A grades 40 years ago. Lubricious Sunday morning sexual intercourse. Back pain severe. More nightmares, Valium notwithstanding. More depression.

7: With Didy to GP Dr. Somers for an examination of her almost healed wounds and cunt. Anger builds in me from where I know not. Dirt everywhere, only menial tasks, amidst small slights, the daily grind. Another huge fight with Didy followed by warmhearted regret.

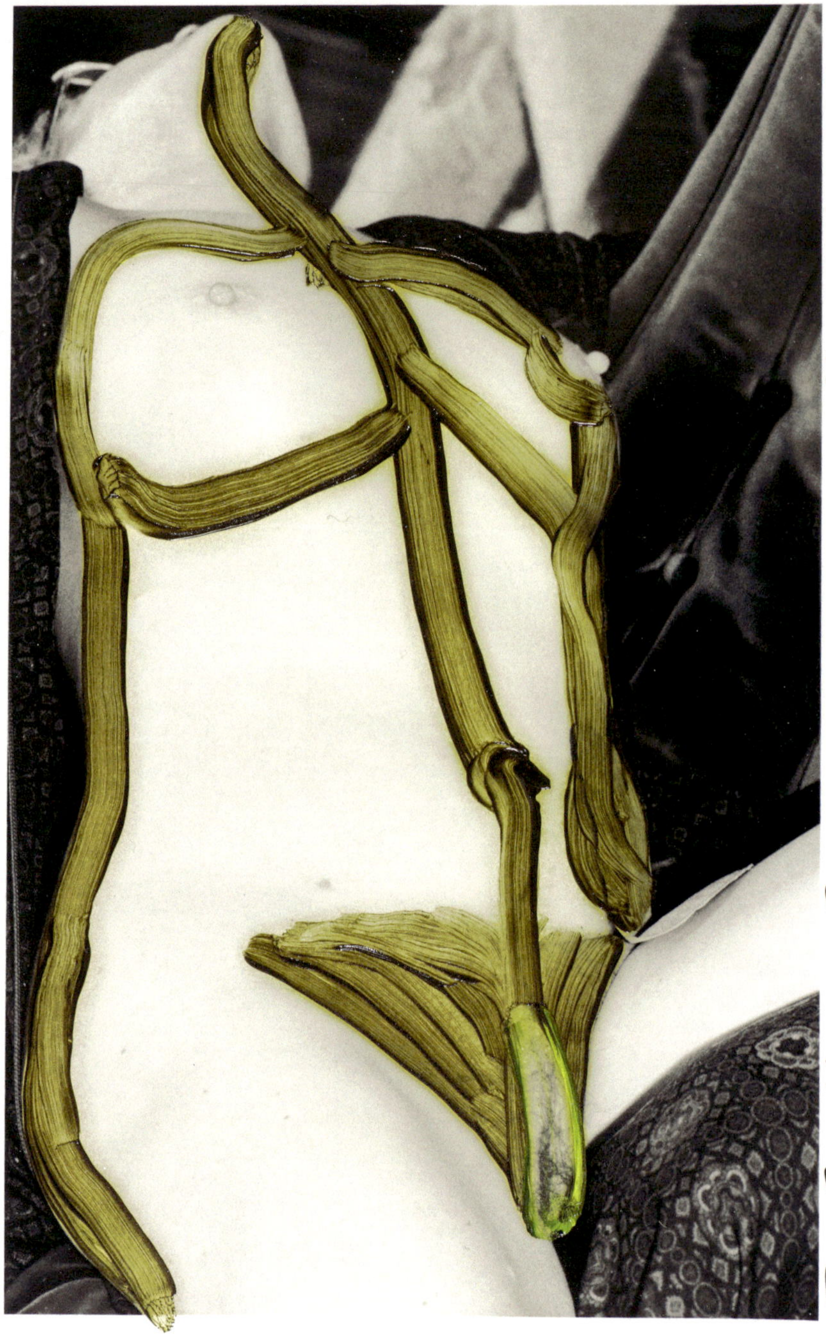

In Red Velvet Chair May 2010

8: Not in a healthy state of mind. Still recovering from fight with Didy which seems to have had no residual effect on her. Wrote letters, drank whiskey, and cooked for Didy. Need to resume photo work soon.

9: Installed new doorbell, inoperative for almost a year. Prepared pasta casserole: roast pork, beets, Chinese veg, and white Italian sauce. Haltingly started to reactivate the darkroom, then started a letter to Geoffrey.

10: Lovely spring day. Still battling an outbreak of genital herpes, a legacy from Susan Rome. This is a component of my depression of course. Finished letter to Geoffrey. Ordered lovely edition of the *Grove Dictionary of Opera*. Finances in good shape.

11: Didy too fatigued to go to the gallery. Garon Awalt for coffee @ 10a. He helped me complete an elegant installation of the exterior Sirius satellite radio antenna. Didy amused by 'men at work'. Then to Pete's for comestibles and wine. Barbeque.

12: Didy to Wolfville with Fran and Wilma for an afternoon's outing. Fran and IJ are trying to cheer up Wilma because her idiot husband abandoned her for a bimbo who will surely leave him.

13: Didy seems to taunt me with slovenly behaviour and careless ways, as if intentionally. She acts as lazy and needy as she says her deceased former partner Mickey was. I suppose that she wants to make damn sure that in this relationship she plays the Mickey part in the drama. Well, I'm grateful to have her notwithstanding that.

14: 4th round of post-operative chemo begins @ 10a with Didy already labouring under extreme fatigue. Appointment with TD Bank investment advisor, who is full of shit. Feeling hopeless and yes, hapless.

15: Chemo @ 8:30a, a brighter day dawns. E-mailed Ellen. Atmosphere in the house improving as chemo comes to an end. Didy looks worse than ever but feels better.

16: Chemo @ 8:30a. Opera: *Nixon in China* (not enamoured of). Made a chicken casserole. I try to cook dishes that will be kind to Didy's delicate chemo up-heaved stomach. Feeling old and worn myself.

17: Chemo @ 1:30p. Didy kissed the head of my swollen cock when we got out of the shower. Strange day, solid letter to Geoffrey. Lovely weather. Cheered by the upcoming end to chemo. An expensive and bad restaurant meal that Didy liked.

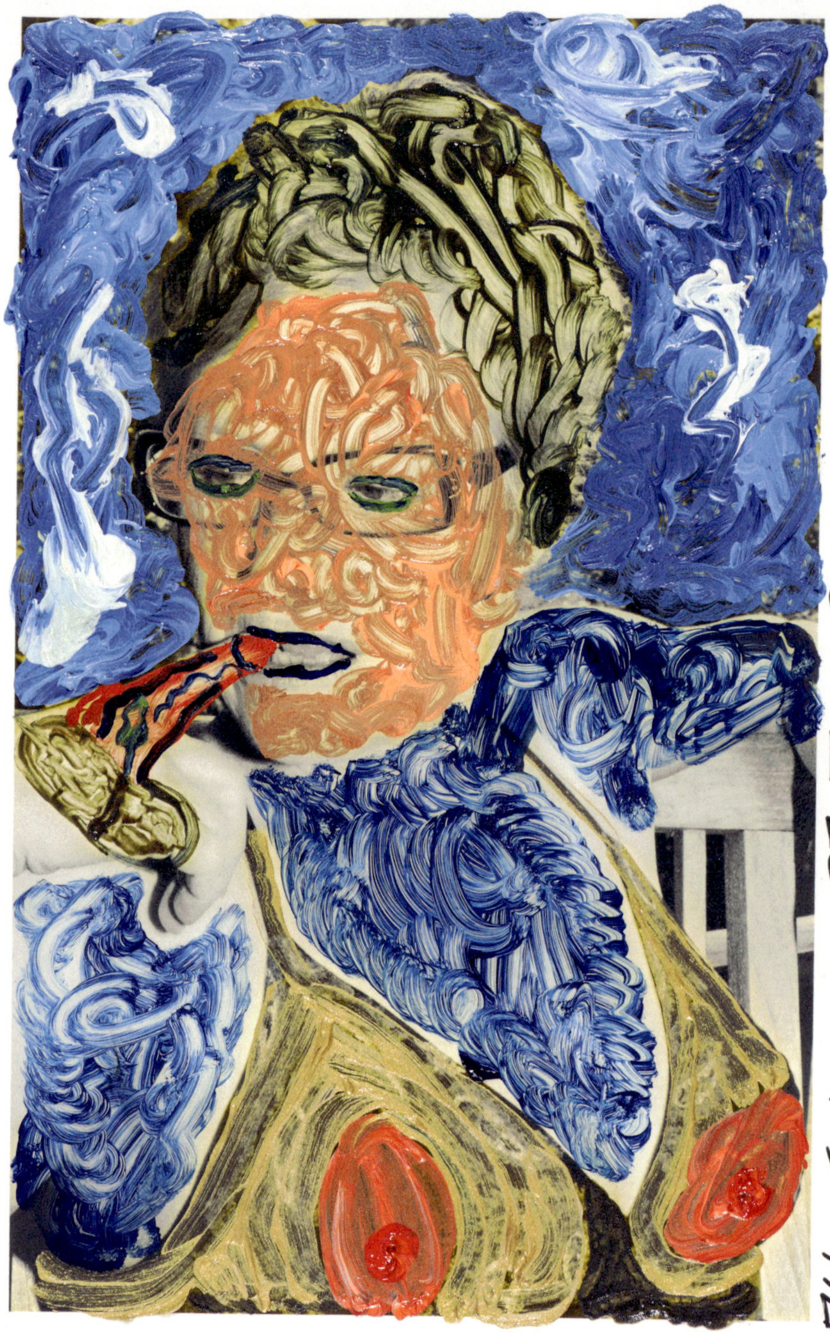

After SEX 27 June 2010

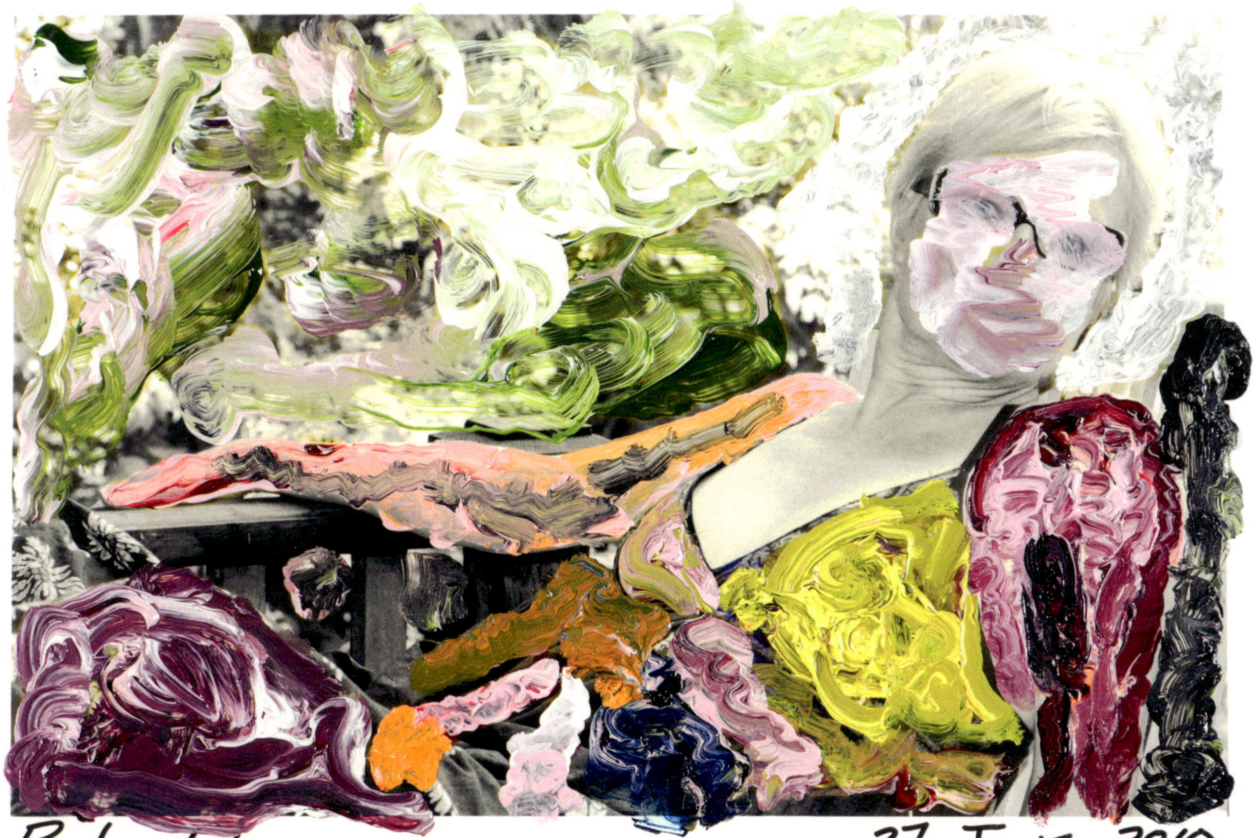

Postcoital 27 June 2010

18: Solid ball-slapping morning sex, then chemo @ 9a. Shopping thereafter, then Didy back to the gallery. A really lovely day. An impromptu party for two to celebrate the end of chemo. Didy difficult, but endearing.

19: Late morning shopping at Pete's. Pleasant afternoon and not too drunk. To Peter and Jayne's for dinner with her Mum. Drove home drunk and carefully @ 12:30p. A happy occasion all round.

20: Slightly hungover. Inclined to have a Cialis tab for a bigger erection. Fucked Didy into a tremorous orgasm. Barbequed prime rib and Portobello mushrooms served with purple asparagus and nice wine.

21: Didy working more hours at the gallery. A sombre day alone, no real work of course, but some household duties accomplished. Getting myself back on the rails is going to take an enormous quantity of inner strength (at the moment depleted).

22: Didy left for the gallery @ 6:45p to smoke in peace I assumed. Very oversexed these days, need something special. Overpriced, and not great, repair to the bathroom tiles.

23: Cleaned the house. Purchased $10K of Precious Metals mutual funds for TFSA. Declined to accompany Didy to Toronto in September for some gatekeepers' conclave. Evolving into a modified self that is unknown to me.

24: Cleaned the house. A dark and dire day that improved with an encounter with Astrid Brunner, not seen since 2008. Didy's car has a slashed tire, replacement ordered. Angry over exploitations. Calmed down with whiskey and a slow-cooked comfort food supper for Didy.

25: Sunny summer morning. Ready to resume house cleaning. Worked on polishing up VW Jetta wagon. Had a few drinks and made a few phone calls with the drinks as fuel.

26: Awake and horny, but Didy was engrossed in a colostomy difficulty. Repeated spontaneous erections all day. Enjoyed Saturday shopping after getting new tire mounted on Didy's car. British Butcher made a great rack of pork. Barbequed of an afternoon.

27: Sunday morning, light streaming in the oversized bedroom window early. Aggressively displayed my cock and balls at the bedside to stimulate Didy's libido. Eventually got her back in bed with "Yes" smeared in lubricant on her labia and my cock's head. Fucked into her hard with Didy squeezing my balls from underneath.

28: Constantly sexually aroused. Letter to Martha & Donigan. Still much housework to do. Losing considerable amount of weight.

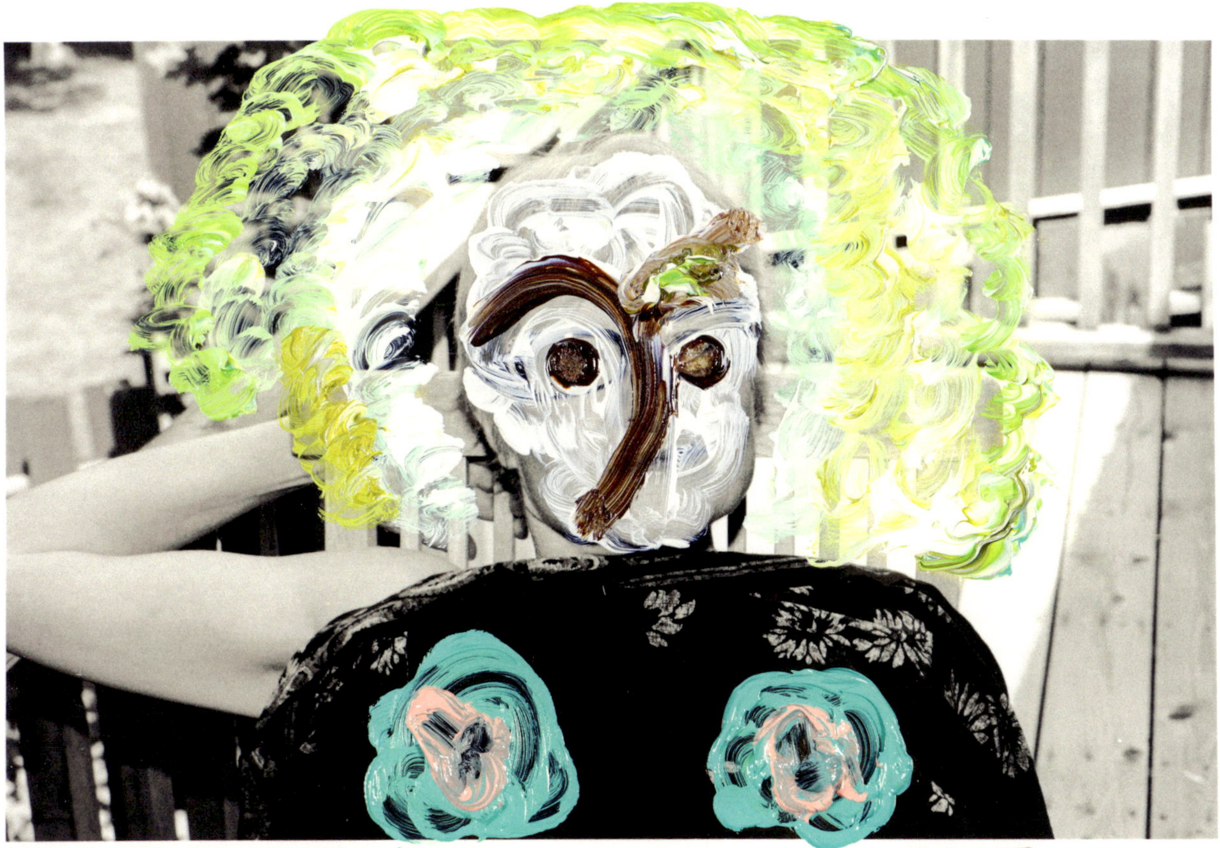

Post-coital tristesse 27 June 2010

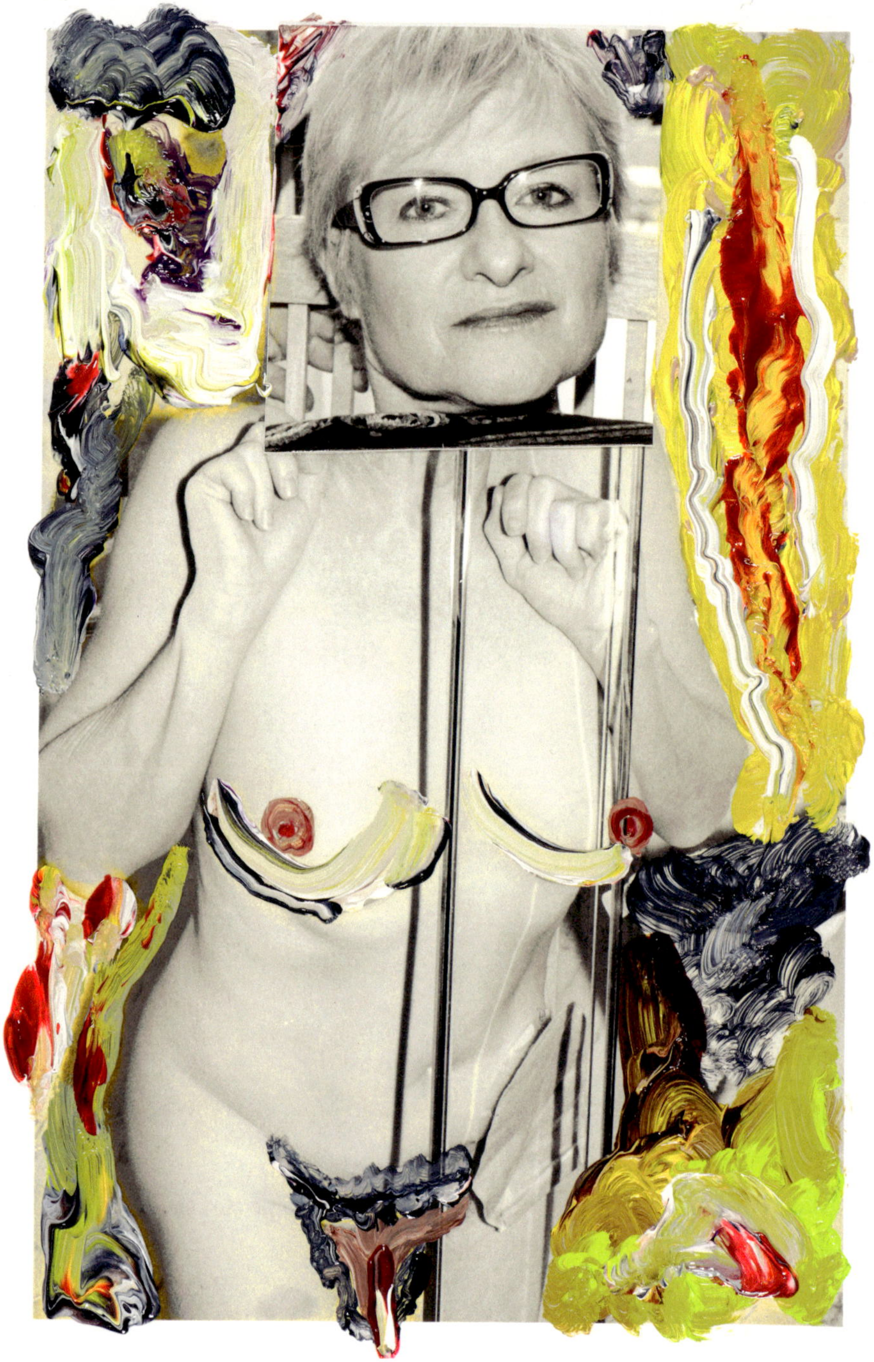

29: Careful and thoughtful letter to Geoffrey S. about his serious problems with his loutish sons. Then made a small potato and Chinese veg casserole. E-mail from an obviously terminally-ill Valerie Dean.

30: Horney and aroused, Didy accepted me with some extravagance and generosity into her lubricated cunt. Return to photo work is relentlessly building. Polished with machinist's cream the '21' brass house number that I designed at the Institute years ago. Thinking of friends all now so far away in time and space.

OCTOBER 2010 (MONTREAL)

22: Bulger to Cat's Inn for a week overlooking Ferguson's Cove. We boarded the Ocean Limited train for the overnight trip to Montreal. Spent a pleasant afternoon in our on-board bedroom, watching the brilliant autumnal coloured landscape go by. Supper in the dining car and a restless night.

23: In Montreal by 9a and to the wonderful Hotel Sofitel on Sherbrooke Street. First viewing of the Otto Dix exhibition at the MMFA. Tremendous! Then to Souvenir Street for a chicken dinner with Martha and Donigan.

24: Slept until 8a, then sloppy penetrative intercourse. Elaborate hotel breakfast and back to the museum for Otto Dix redux. Took a break in the hotel room for drinks then back to other shows at the MMFA. Sumptuous hotel dinner with an excellent Sancerre.

25: Sex in the middle of the night with Didy riding. Donigan phoned to make plans for tomorrow. Out in the rain for coffee and whiskey shopping. Then walked to Schwartz's Deli for huge pastrami sandwiches. Back at the hotel, shot Didy nude in the glass shower with the fisheye lens. Watched TV with whiskey.

26: Morning coffee together, IJ off to her conference and I walked to Souvenir Street for an important meeting of the old 'Souvenir Club'—Martha, Donigan, and myself. Confidences proffered and exchanged. Silently bid goodbye to 'Doc', the dying golden retriever. Dinner with Martha, Donigan, and Didy in my old territory on St. Denis at a very Francophone hipster bistro (formerly the beloved Witloof Belgian restaurant).

27: Intercourse with Didy spread-legged and upright on the edge of the bathroom vanity. Post-coital photographs. Packed up for the trip home. One last viewing of the Otto Dix. Then shopping at Holt-Renfrew for cashmere items for Didy. Waited in the hotel bar for Didy to return from the conference, then an exciting Montreal-style mad-dash cab ride to the Gare Centrale.

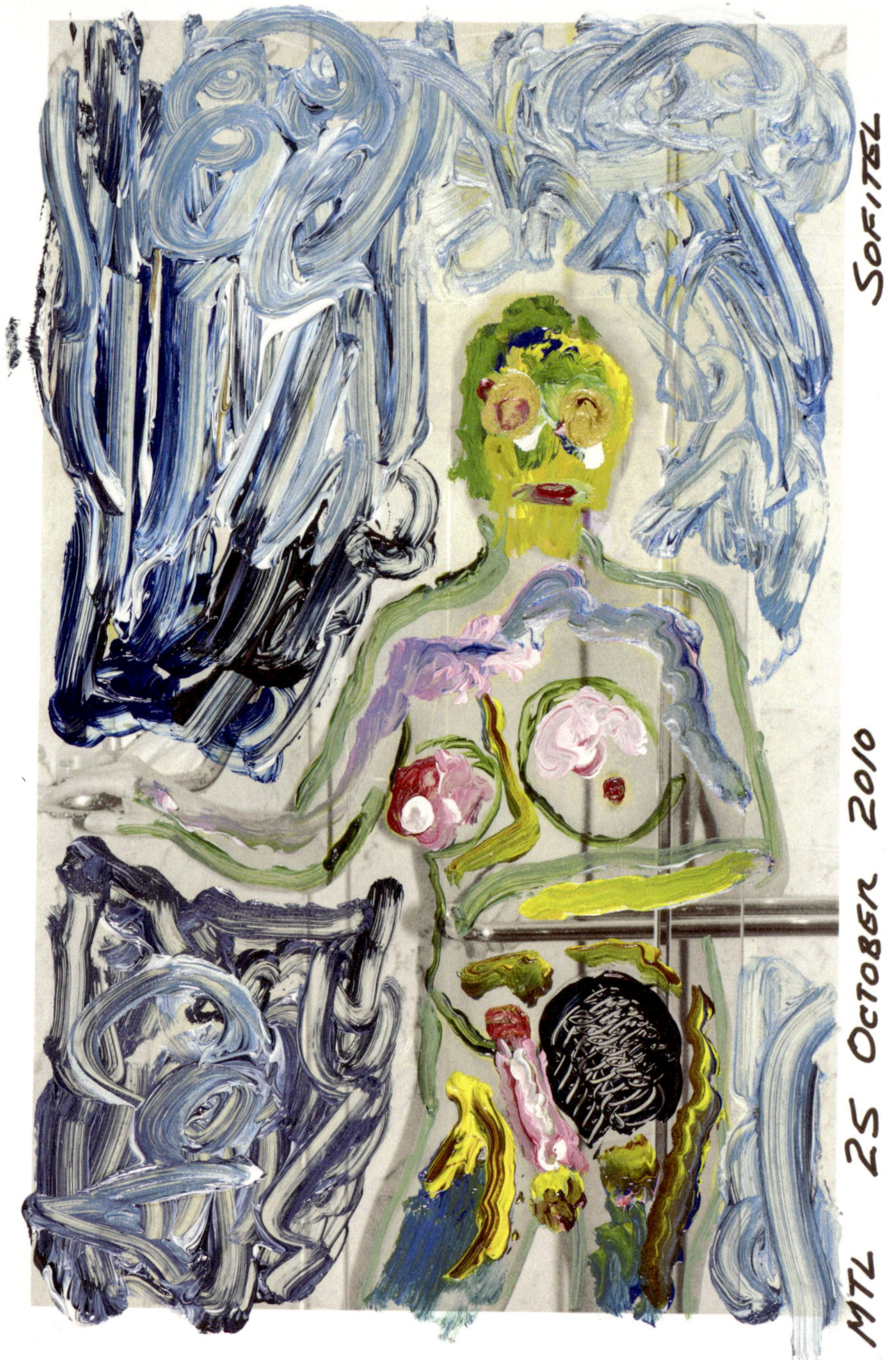
Sofitel
MTL 25 October 2010

28: On the train all night and most of the day. Very spectacular landscapes, colours, and atmospheric lighting effects all the way to Halifax. Didy intended to read, but instead watched the passing scenes and sipped whiskey. Always grand to return home to the photo-bunker. Didy upbeat and enthused by the little trip to Montreal.

29: Bailed the Bulger out of the cat hotel, where she totally charmed the proprietress. She's delighted to be home. Worked up family accounts, spent $6K this month. Made beef & pasta casserole while Didy went to officiate at a 'Beauty Pageant.'

DECEMBER 2010 (BERLIN)

23: 2nd wedding anniversary. Festive day of pre-trip celebrating and a slow burning buildup to sexual consummation. Delivered the Bulger to the seaside cat hotel. Pre-packing, trip organizing, then out for Japanese meal. Middle of the night frantic sex.

24: Christmas Eve Day. Halifax to Ottawa, then Ottawa to Frankfurt (departed 5:00p).

25: Christmas Day. Arrived in Frankfurt and departed @ 10:25a for Berlin, arrived at Tegel airport @ 11:30 a. Then by cab to Charlottenburg and the pre-war Hotel Astoria at Fasanenstraße 2. Settled into a top floor room overlooking a parking lot with large bronze statues. A prearranged Christmas dinner at the Berlin Plaza: smoked fish and salad, giblet soup, pheasant breast with pineapple sauerkraut & potato dumplings. Dear Wolfgang phoned us from Canada, so excited to talk to us in Berlin.

26: Sunday. To the Berliner Dom in the sunshine and fresh snow for full Lutheran service with communion (Festgottesdienst mit Abendmahl) @ 10a. Moved to tears by the beauty of an old believers' church service with superb choir, organist, and solo trumpeter. Thoughts of childhood as the familiar hymns brought back memories. After the service crossed the Unter den Linden to the opulent Operncafé for a traditional and extensive German Sunday lunch.

27: Monday. Tramped around Charlottenburg in the snow. Photographed all day with refuelling stops for schnaps (Williams Birne). Ate at the great Berlin department store KaDeWe: potato pancakes, blood sausage, and dark beer. Shopped for Didy: La Perla lingerie, fancy red woollen hat with feathers, and then a cashmere sweater while going out the door.

28: Tuesday. Gemäldegalerie (Picture Gallery) on Museum Island, amazingly beautiful neoclassical bullet-ridden façade; *Hommage an Caravaggio* was featured, though the permanent collection was astounding. Museum guardians looked like re-purposed GDR prison wardens. Lunched at the legendary Dressler restaurant on Unter den Linden, where one can easily imagine an SS staff car parked outside. Of an evening, to the

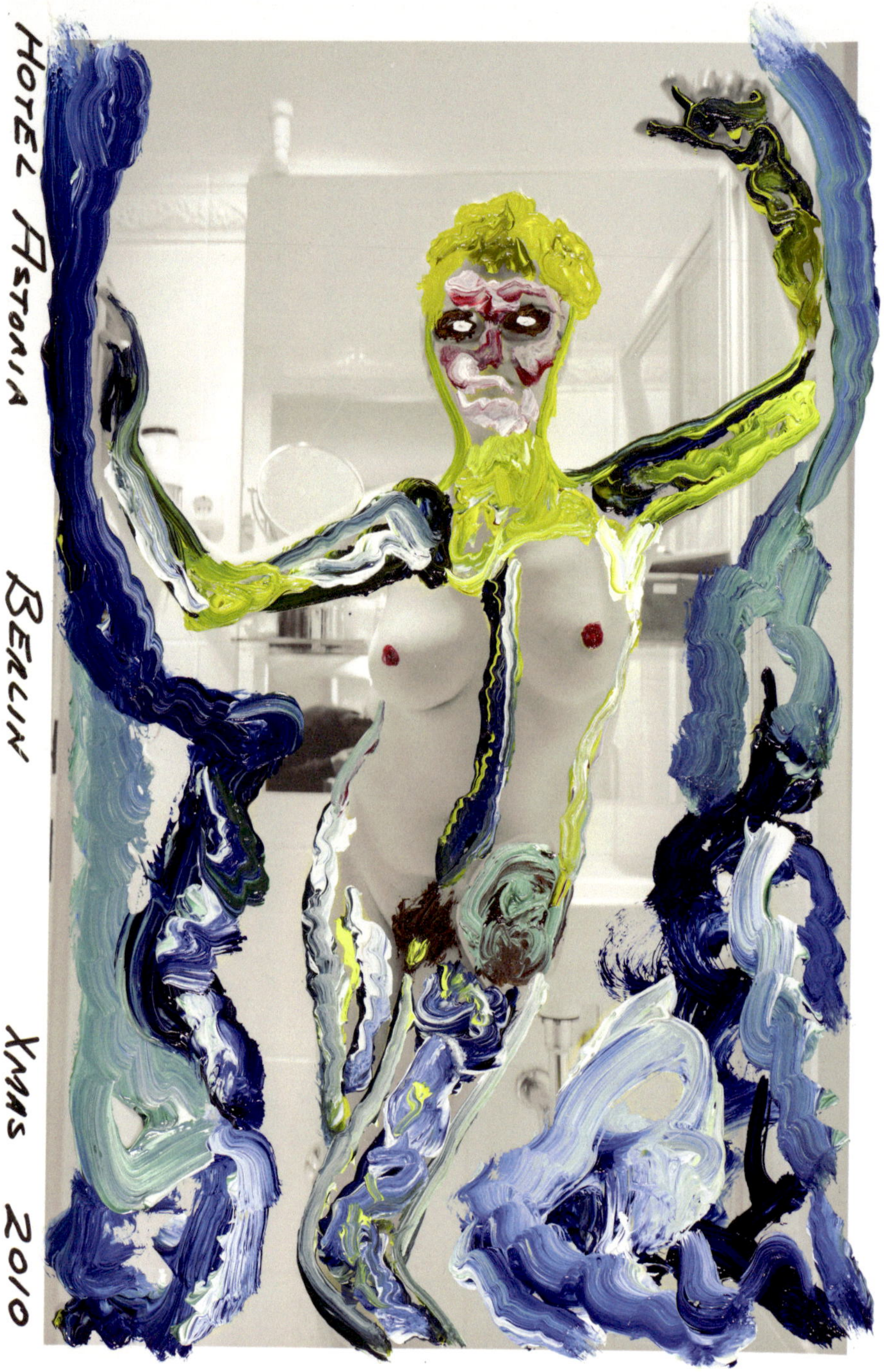
HOTEL ASTORIA BERLIN XMAS 2010

Staatsoper im Schiller Theater for a delightful performance of Mozart's *Die Zauberflöte*. Walked through the snowy streets, arm in arm, back to the hotel with its questionable wartime pedigree.

29: Wednesday. Pergamonmuseum, awed by the Pergamon Altar, the Ishtar Gate, and the Market Gate of Miletus. A museum experience like no other. Elegant late lunch at Galeries Lafayette, for me the oysters followed by fish broth. Deutsche Oper Berlin, Bismarckstraße 35, for *La Traviata*. Didy sat next to an elegant Japanese lady, both cried extensively. After the performance, staggered back to the Astoria for schnaps purchased at the Dicke Wirtin for in-room drinking.

30: Thursday. Berlinische Galerie, for the Nan Goldin retrospective photo show. A pleasant lunch at the gallery, then explored its upper floor and discovered Albert Speer's original scale model of Welthauptstadt (World Capital) Germania. Back to the Staatsoper im Schiller Theater for Mozart's *Così Fan Tutte,* a sprightly near perfect-pitch production set in the 1950s.

31: New Year's Eve. Dinner of Berliner specialties at the Knese restaurant; I had knuckle of pork, crisply fried and served on a bed of malt beer sauce with Bavarian cabbage and bread dumplings. Walked slowly back to the hotel in the falling snow. Crossed the Kurfürstendamm boulevard where the snowy trees were covered in white lights and then turned up Fasanenstraße arm in arm and chatting to ourselves. The New Year's Eve fireworks could be heard in the distance probably in the Tiergarten, creating a wartime rather than festive atmosphere. Suddenly a German policeman with an automatic carbine across his chest appeared beside us out of the shadows. We were speechless with shock, but continued on at a steady pace. Later I realized that the policeman was guarding the site of the Fasanenstraße Synagoge, burned during Kristallnacht in 1938 and destroyed by the Royal Air Force in 1943. Photographed Didy nude in our tiny bathroom at the Hotel Astoria. For the long exposure times required, I improvised a camera support using a wooden chair on top of a coffee table. Departed in the morning for Venice via Munich.

Epilogue

> The intellect of man is forced to choose
> perfection of the life, or of the work,
> And if it take the second must refuse
> A heavenly mansion, raging in the dark.
> When all that story's finished, what's the news?
> In luck or out the toil has left its mark:
> That old perplexity an empty purse,
> Or the day's vanity, the night's remorse.
>
> —WILLIAM BUTLER YEATS

It is now 2017, seven years have passed after the events herein described and depicted. Ingrid is still alive; her cancer has not returned. We are still together. We have aged far more than would be expected.

The journey through Cancerland did not stop when this work did. It continues to this day. Little is said by either of us. We both know what the stakes are. One adapts to living with heightened uncertainty, and its ever present peril. It's hard to say if this amplifies perceptions or grinds them down through suppression. The former, I'd say.

Of course, there have been other hard realities for us to face in the intervening seven years. The process of forging a marriage that is anchored in the experience of cancer has continued as a perpetual and difficult work-in-progress. The summer after Ingrid's treatment was over, we installed all around the house an extensive formal garden to which she is fervently devoted. We have collaborated on several exhibition projects for Ingrid's gallery. Every autumn we travel to Europe for music, art, and history, always grateful to escape the North American repression. Ingrid's beloved father Wolfgang has died. We both feel his absence keenly. Certain predictable and some unexpected physical afflictions have come upon us. I suffered a minor stroke in 2013. The darkroom, though, is still in full operation. Our world, as expected, is thinning and dimming.

Dramatis Personae

IJ (Didy)	Ingrid Jenkner, wife of George Steeves
GS	George Steeves
Mickey	Arthur Handy (d. 2004), former spouse of Ingrid
Karin	Karin Jenkner, younger sister of Ingrid
Wolfgang	father of Ingrid and Karin (d. 2015)
Elders	Wolfgang and his wife, mother of Ingrid and Karin
Helen	mother (d. 2005) of GS
Aubrey	father (d. 2000) of GS
Judith	sister of GS
Linda	Linda Payzant (née Toy), 1st wife (1964–78) of GS
NSR	Norah Susan Rome, 2nd wife (1986–96) of GS
Miss Heller (LFH)	Liane Frances Heller, lover and model (1997–2007) of GS
Susanna Heller	sister of Liane
Angela	Angela Lane (née Holloway), lover and model (1984–85) of GS
Ellen	Ellen Pierce, lover and model (1981–83) of GS
Richard Simmins	friend (d.1999) of GS
Marjorie Simmins	daughter of Richard
Geoffrey Simmins	son of Richard
Martha	Martha Langford, staunch supporter and friend of GS
Donigan (DTC)	Donigan Cumming, husband of Martha and friend of GS
Chester Pelkey	friend (d. 2012) of GS
Garon	Garon Awalt, engineering colleague and shipmate of GS
Valerie Dean	dear friend and model of GS, died of colon cancer 2011
Peter Dykhuis & Jayne Wark	friends of Ingrid and then of George
Peggy	Peggy MacKinnon, Ingrid's capable second in command at the gallery.

Acknowledgements

Dr. Astrid Brunner
Donigan Cumming
Dr. Martha Langford
Reverend Dr. Geoffrey Simmins

Published by
Studio George Steeves
21 Tangmere Crescent
Halifax, Canada B3M 1K2
e-mail: georgesteeves@ns.sympatico.ca

Designed by Robert Tombs, Ottawa
Printed by Lowe-Martin, Ottawa
Bound by Multi Bookbinding, Shawinigan

LIBRARY AND ARCHIVES CANADA
CATALOGUING IN PUBLICATION

Steeves, George, author, photographer
Excision / George Steeves.

ISBN 978-0-9959833-0-4 (hardcover)

1. Jenkner, Ingrid, 1955- —Health. 2. Steeves, George.
3. Colon (Anatomy)—Cancer—Patients—Biography. I. Title.

RC280.C6S74 2017 616.99'43470092 C2017-903998-9